©

Copyright 2022 - All rights reserved.

You may not reproduce, duplicate or send the contents of this book without direct written permission from the author. You cannot apply hereby despite any circumstance blame the publisher or hold him or her to legal responsibility for any reparation, compensations, or monetary forfeiture owing to the information included herein, either in a direct or an indirect way.

Legal Notice: This book has copyright protection. You can use the book for personal purposes. You should not sell, use, alter, distribute, quote, take excerpts, or paraphrase in part or whole the material contained in this book without obtaining the permission of the author first.

Disclaimer Notice: You must take note that the information in this document is for casual reading and entertainment purposes only. We have made every attempt to provide accurate, up-to-date, and reliable information. We do not express or imply guarantees of any kind. The persons who read admit that the writer is not occupied in giving legal, financial, medical, or other advice. We put this book content by sourcing various places.

Please consult a licensed professional before you try any techniques shown in this book. By going through this document, the book lover comes to an an agreement that under no situation is the author accountable for any forfeiture, direct or indirect, which they may incur because of the use of material contained in this document, including, but not limited to, — errors, omissions, or inaccuracies.

Shooting Log Book

Belongs to

_____
_____
_____

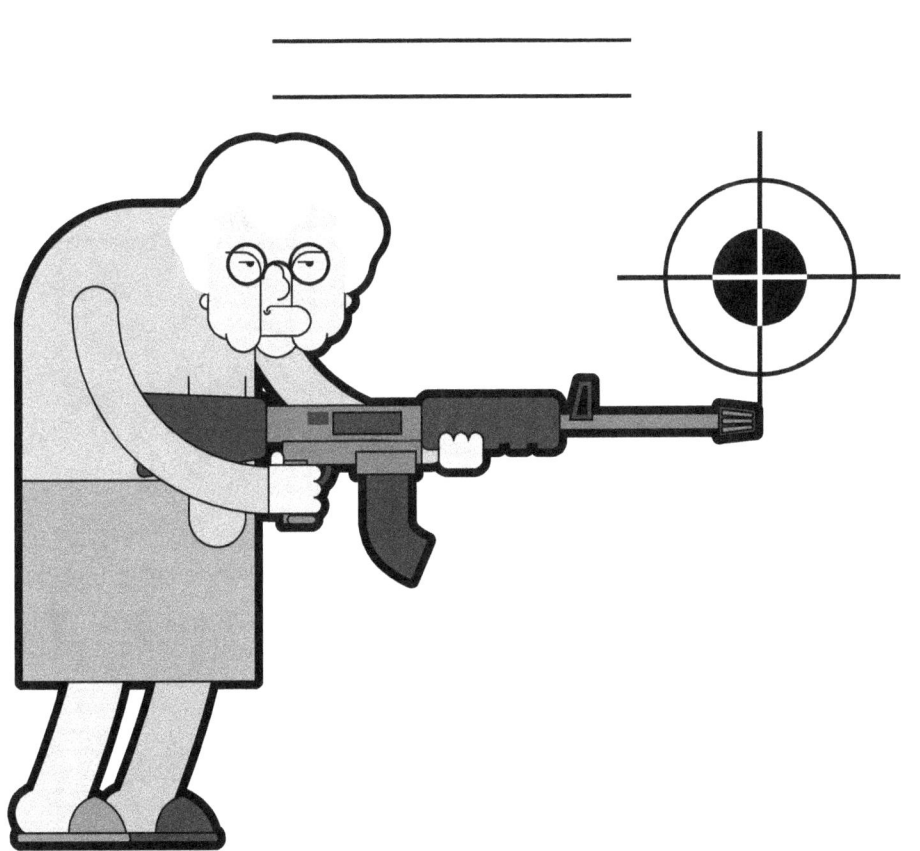

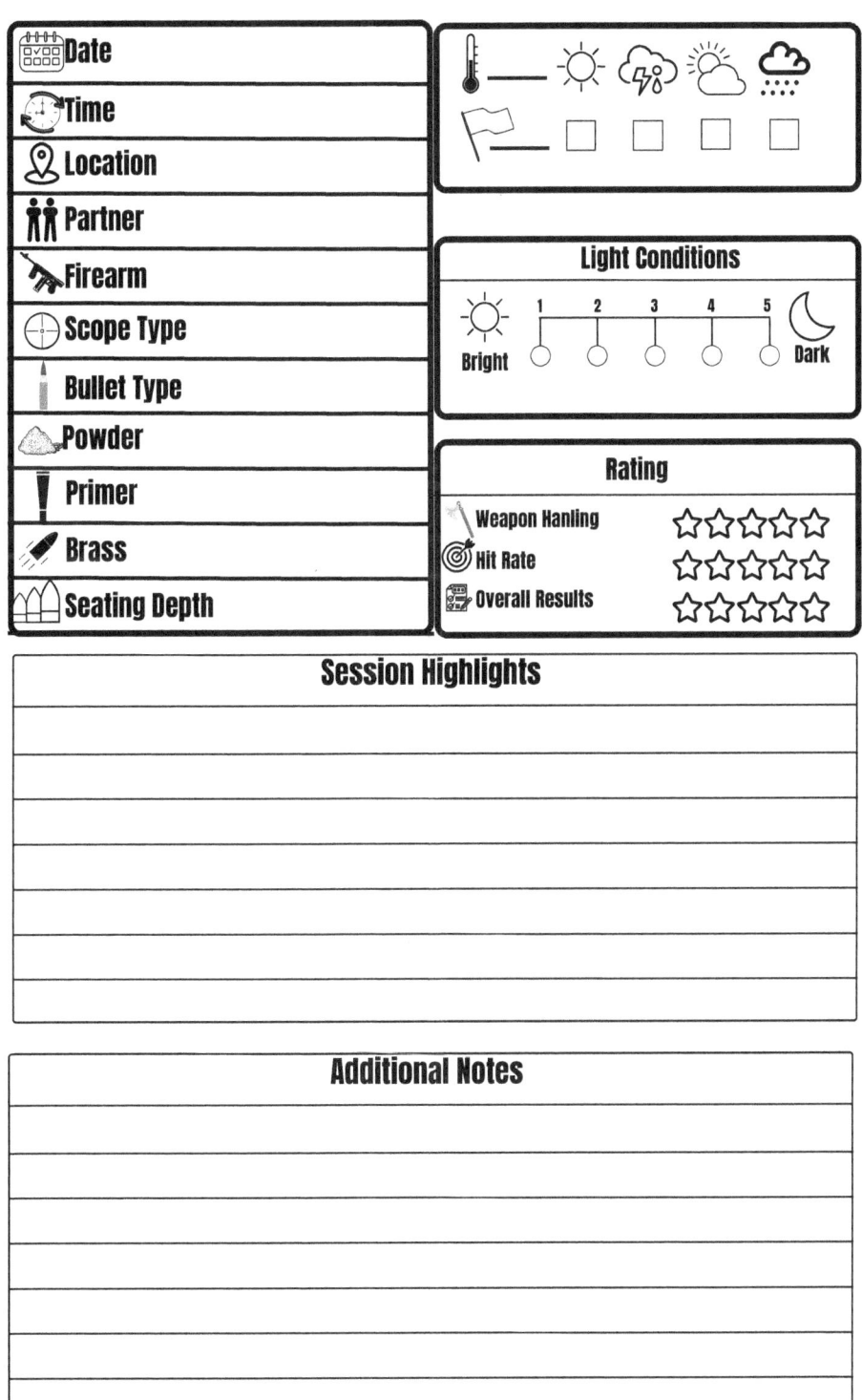

Session Highlights

Additional Notes

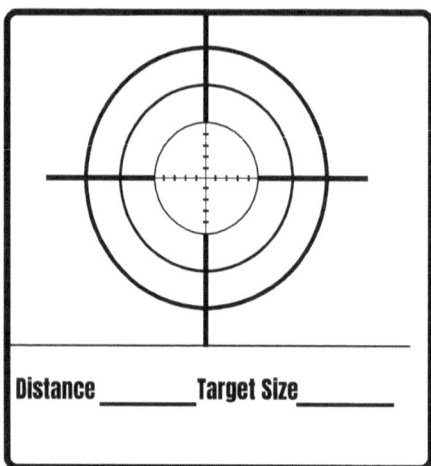
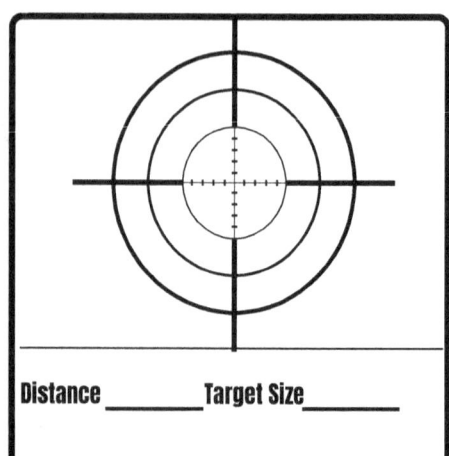
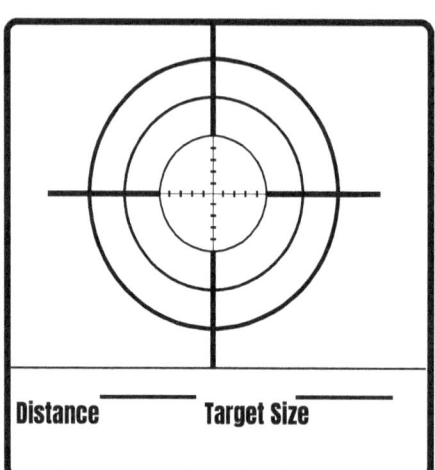
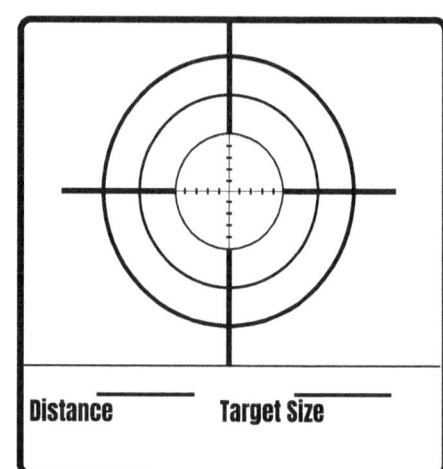
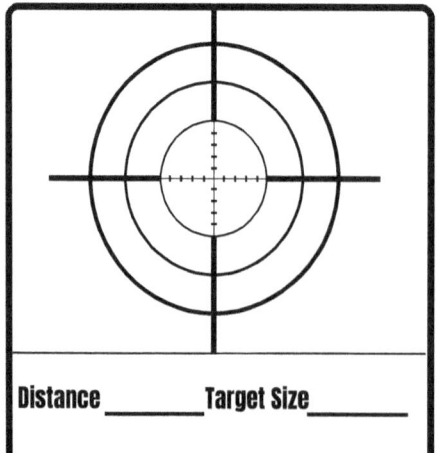
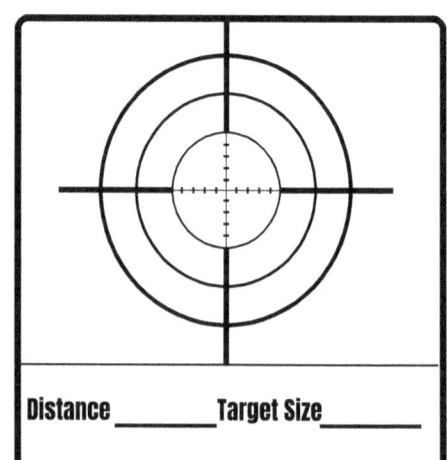

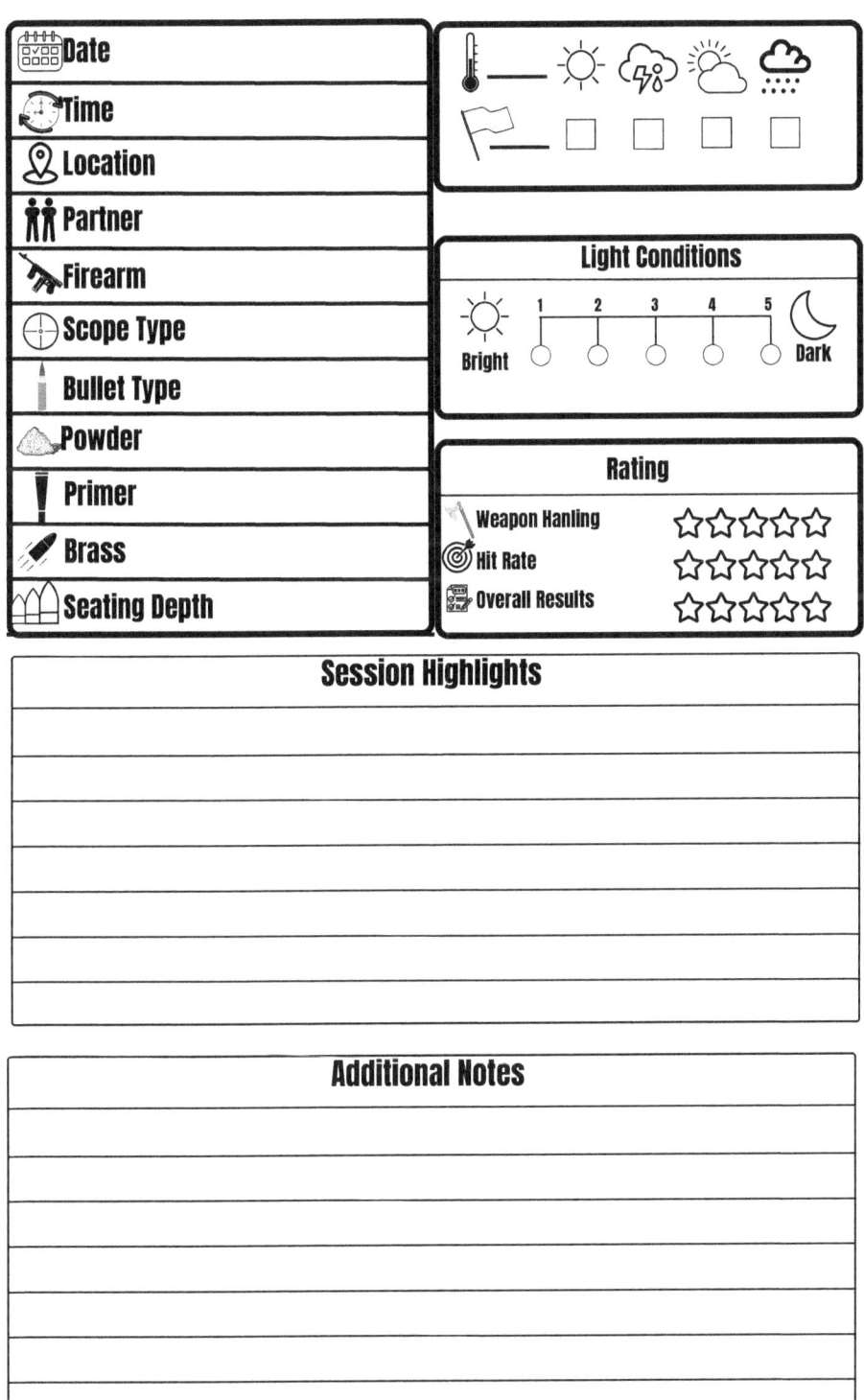

Date	
Time	
Location	
Partner	
Firearm	
Scope Type	
Bullet Type	
Powder	
Primer	
Brass	
Seating Depth	

Light Conditions

Bright 1 2 3 4 5 Dark

Rating

Weapon Hanling	☆☆☆☆☆
Hit Rate	☆☆☆☆☆
Overall Results	☆☆☆☆☆

Session Highlights

Additional Notes

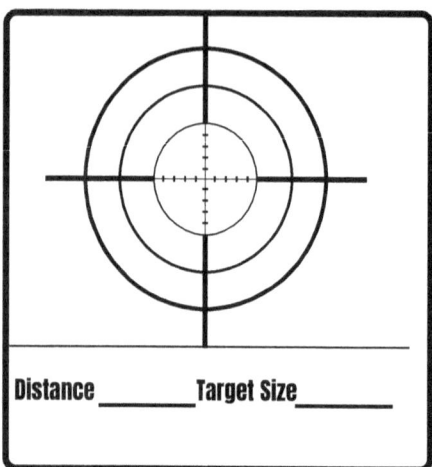

Distance _____ Target Size _____

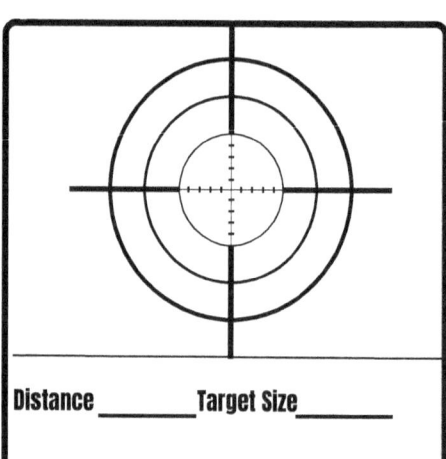

Distance _____ Target Size _____

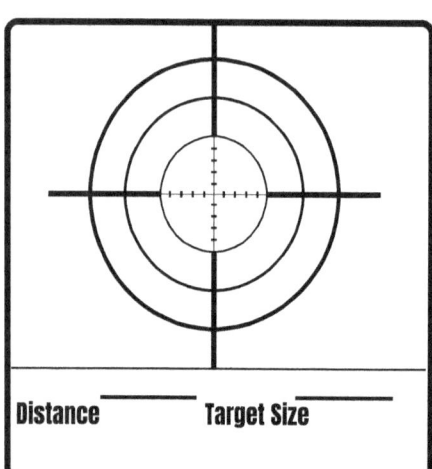

Distance _____ Target Size _____

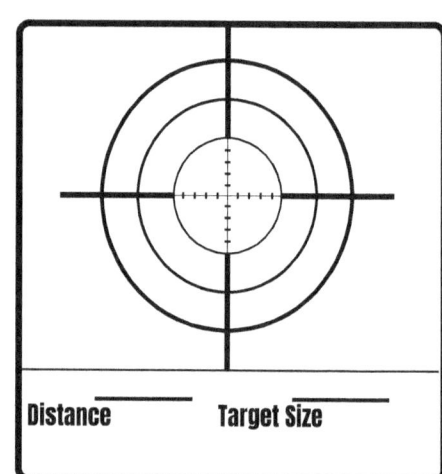

Distance _____ Target Size _____

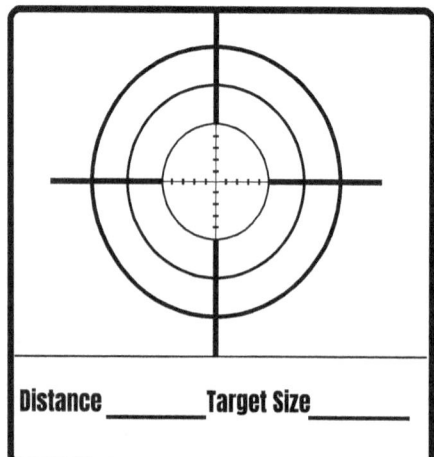

Distance _____ Target Size _____

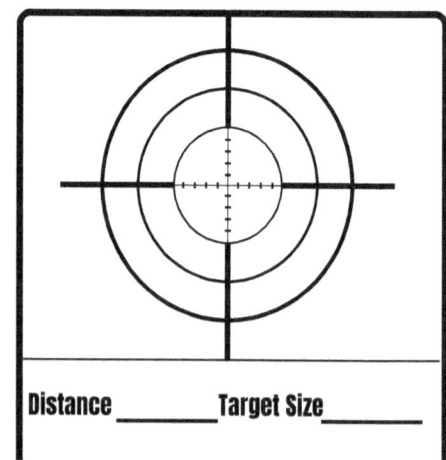

Distance _____ Target Size _____

- Date
- Time
- Location
- Partner
- Firearm
- Scope Type
- Bullet Type
- Powder
- Primer
- Brass
- Seating Depth

Light Conditions

Bright 1 — 2 — 3 — 4 — 5 Dark

Rating

- Weapon Hanling ☆☆☆☆☆
- Hit Rate ☆☆☆☆☆
- Overall Results ☆☆☆☆☆

Session Highlights

Additional Notes

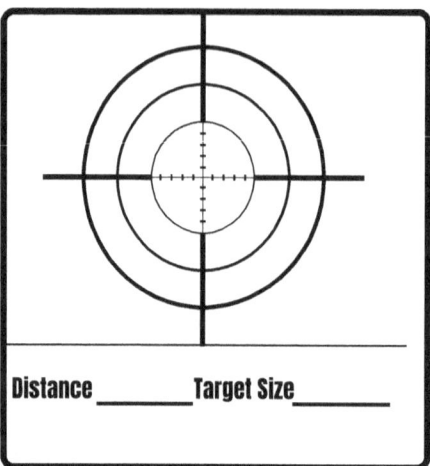

Distance _____ Target Size _____

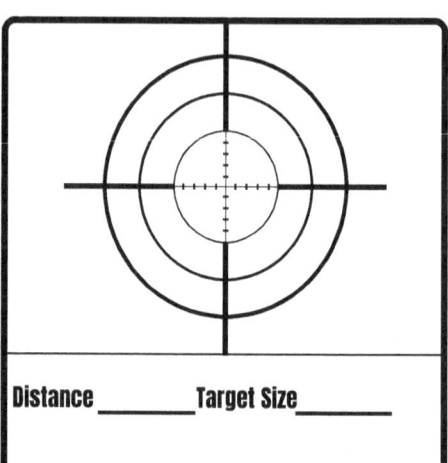

Distance _____ Target Size _____

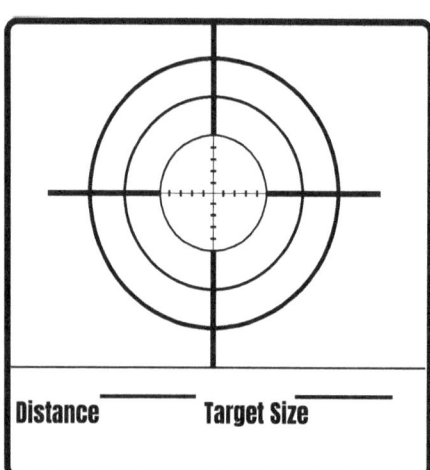

Distance _____ Target Size _____

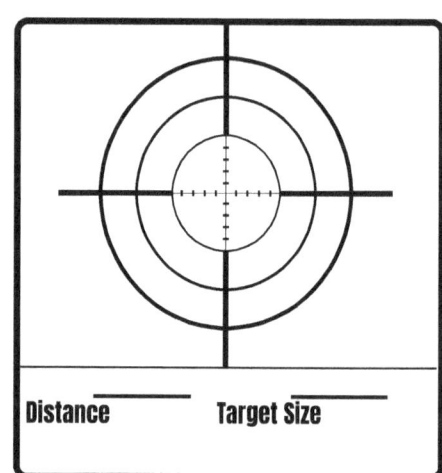

Distance _____ Target Size _____

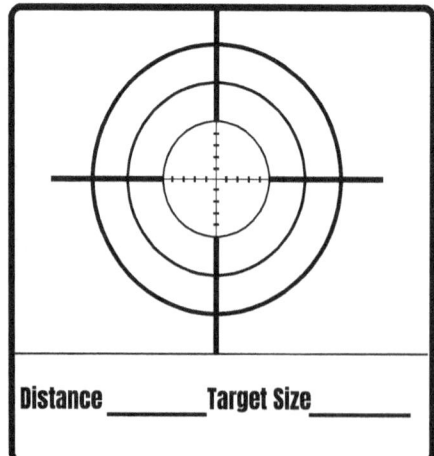

Distance _____ Target Size _____

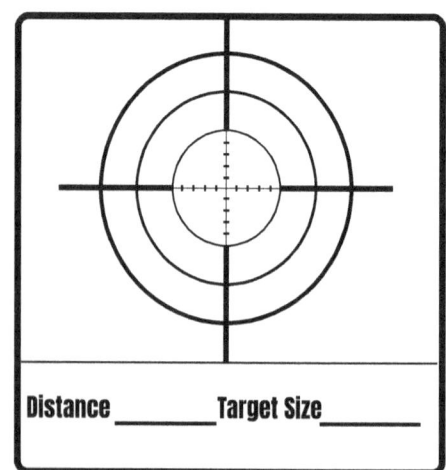

Distance _____ Target Size _____

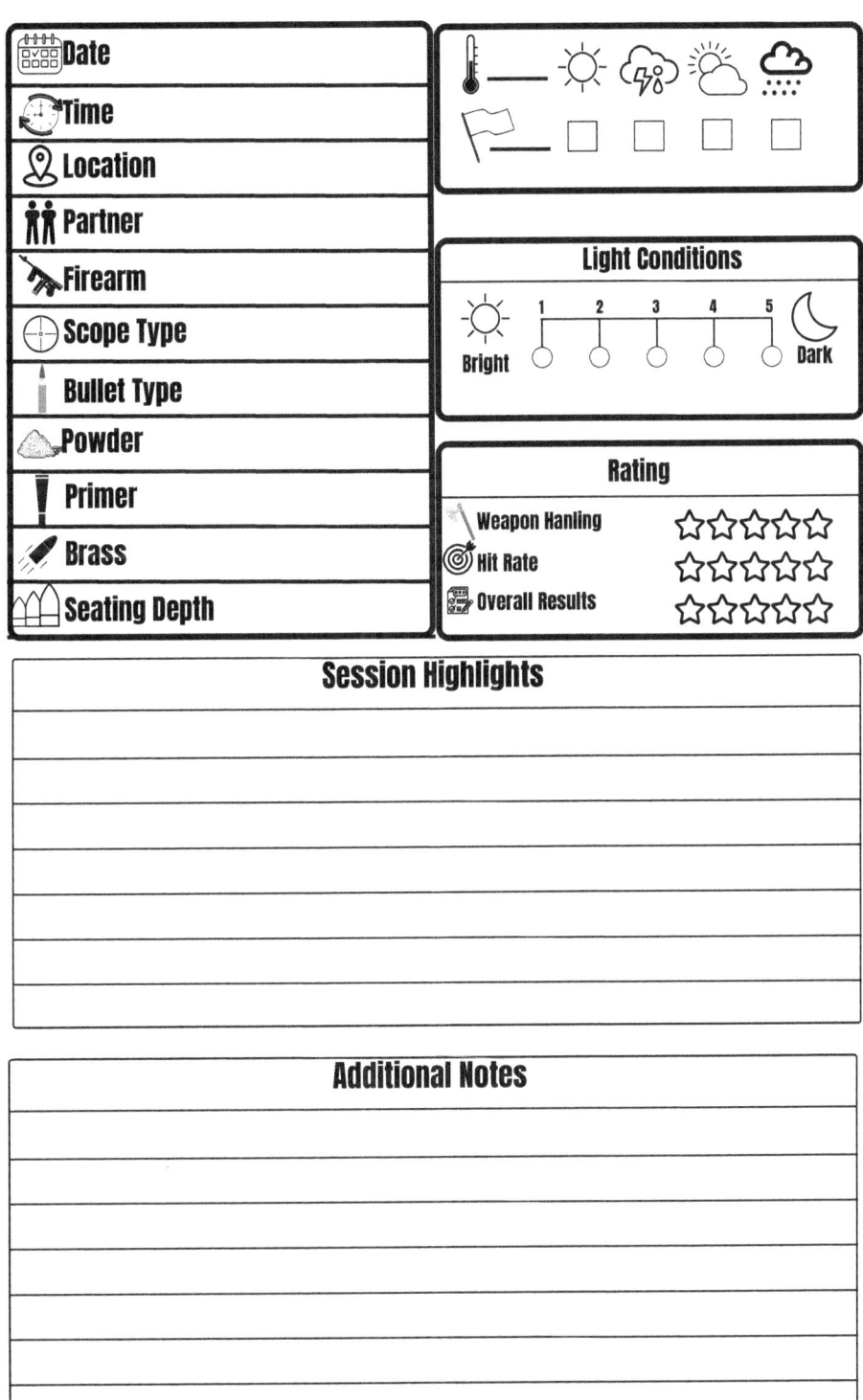

Date	
Time	
Location	
Partner	
Firearm	
Scope Type	
Bullet Type	
Powder	
Primer	
Brass	
Seating Depth	

Light Conditions

Bright 1 2 3 4 5 Dark

Rating

- Weapon Hanling ☆☆☆☆☆
- Hit Rate ☆☆☆☆☆
- Overall Results ☆☆☆☆☆

Session Highlights

Additional Notes

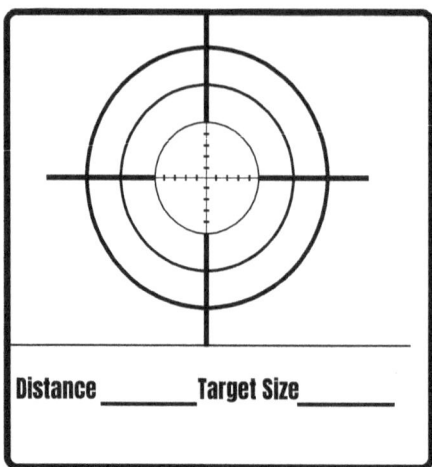

Distance_____ Target Size_____

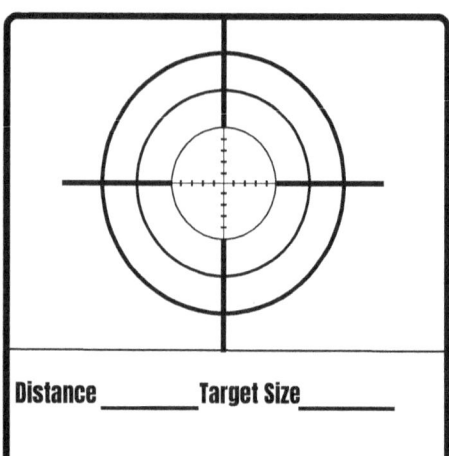

Distance_____ Target Size_____

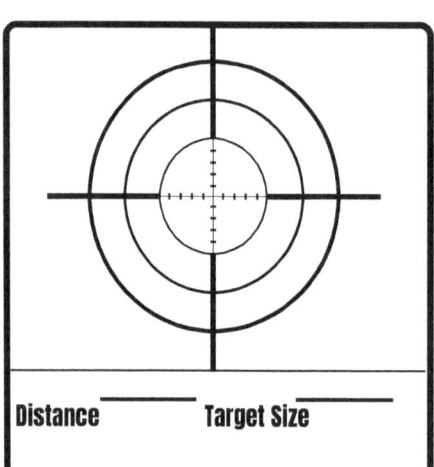

Distance_____ Target Size_____

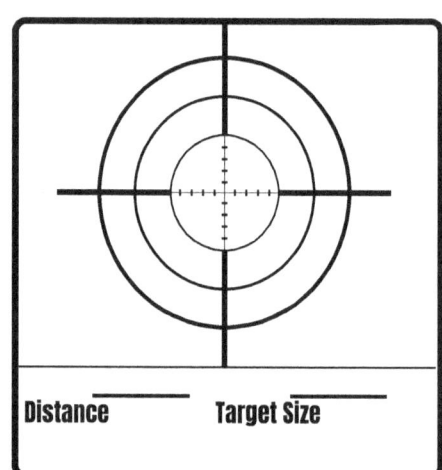

Distance_____ Target Size_____

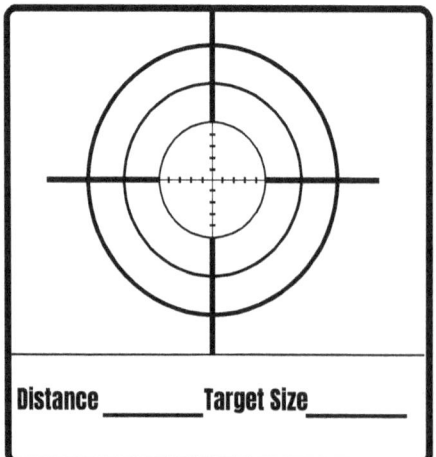

Distance_____ Target Size_____

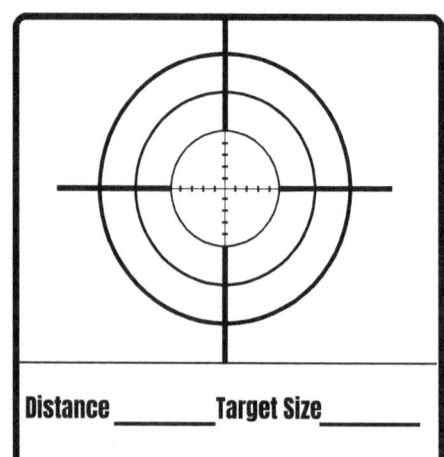

Distance_____ Target Size_____

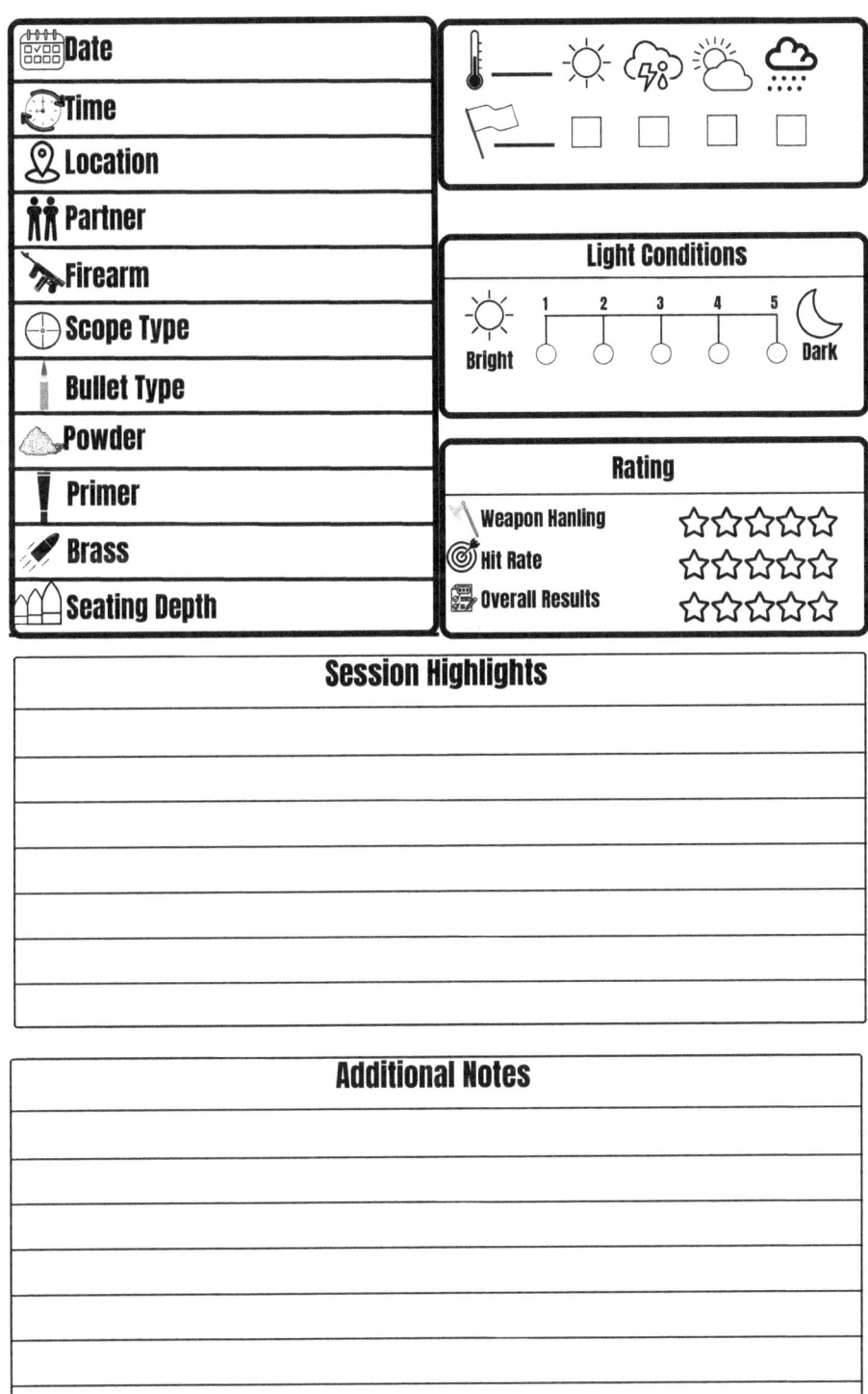

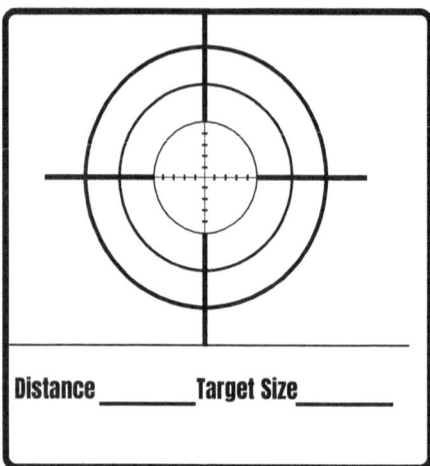
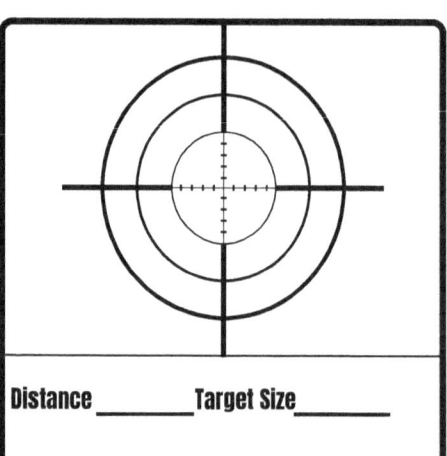
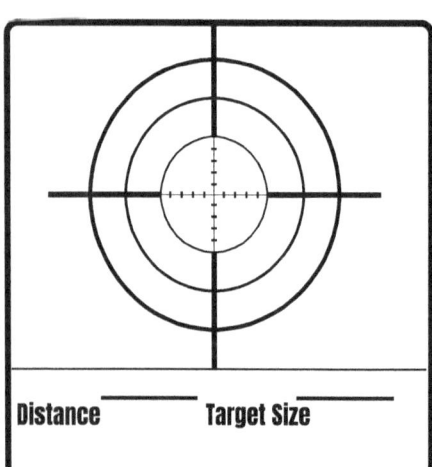
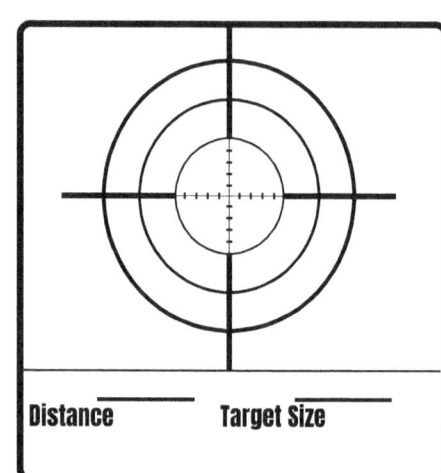
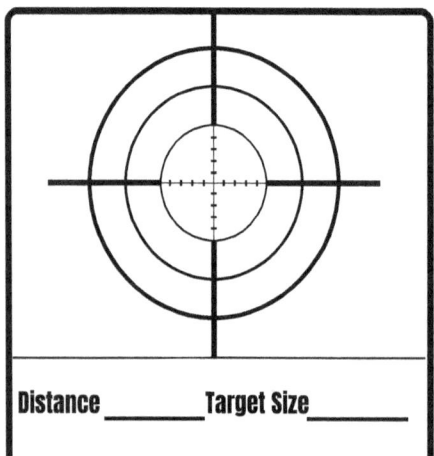
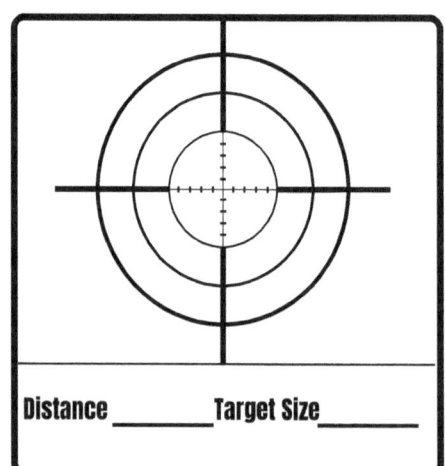

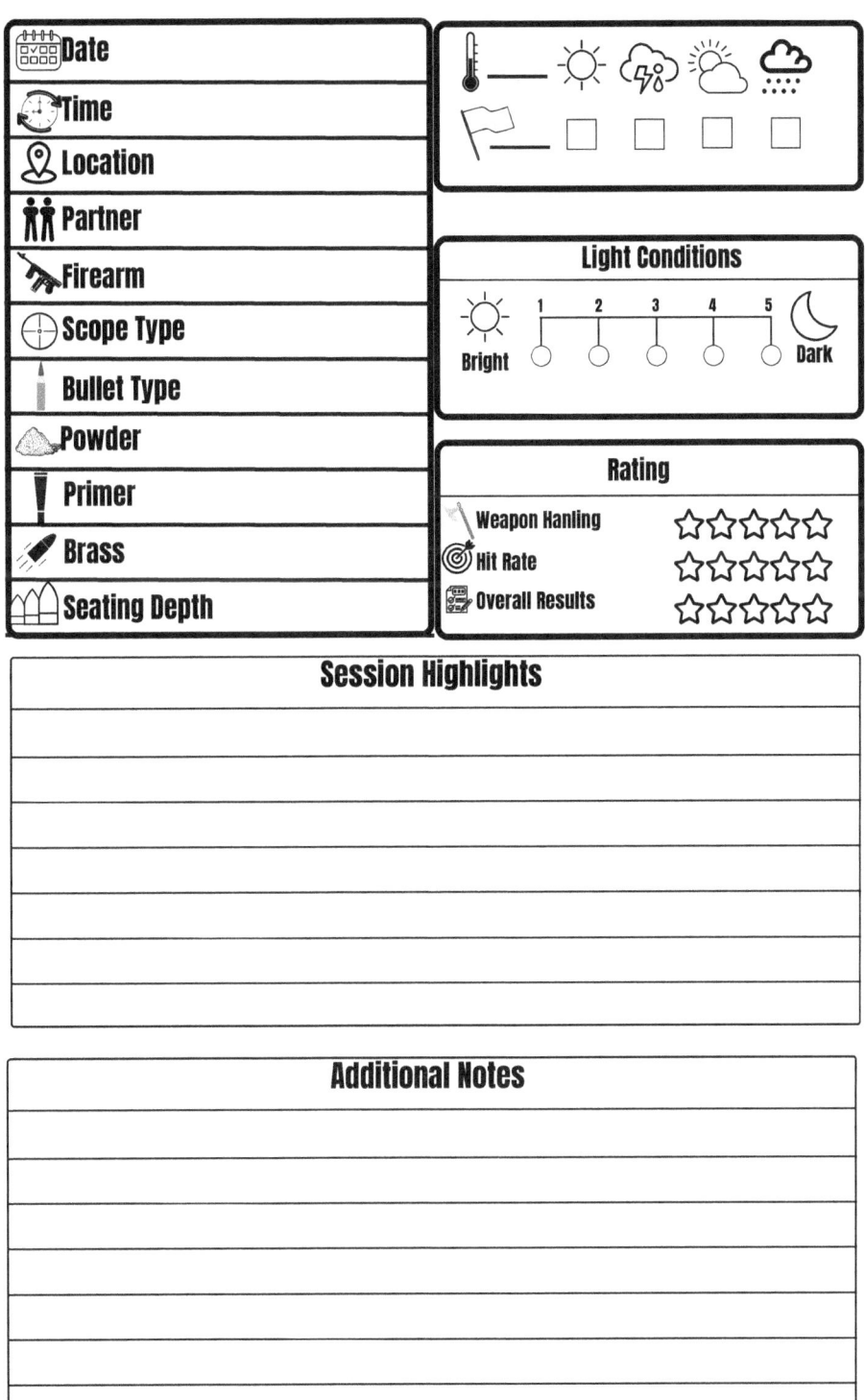

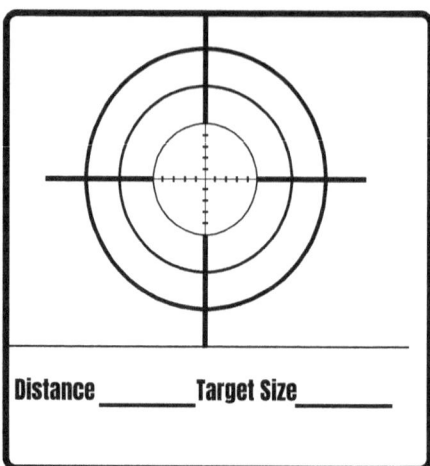

Distance _____ Target Size _____

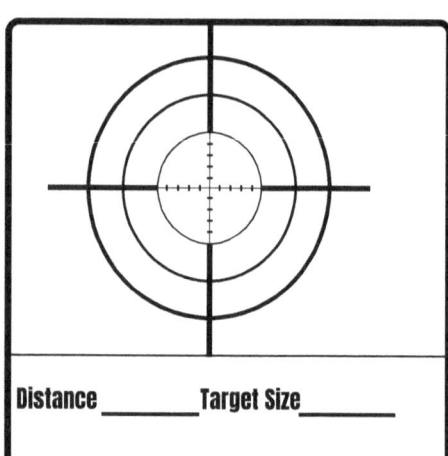

Distance _____ Target Size _____

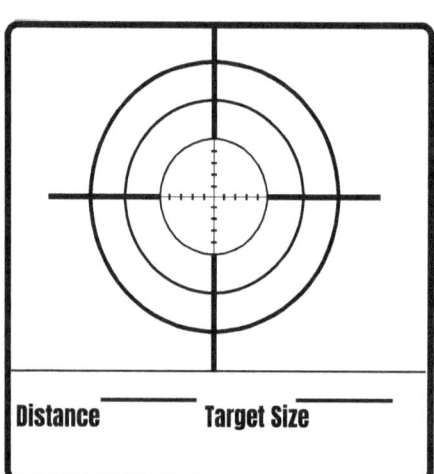

Distance _____ Target Size _____

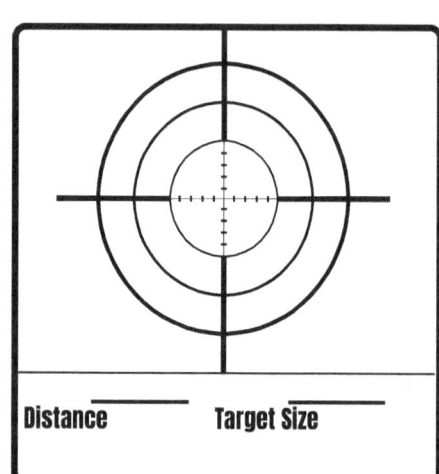

Distance _____ Target Size _____

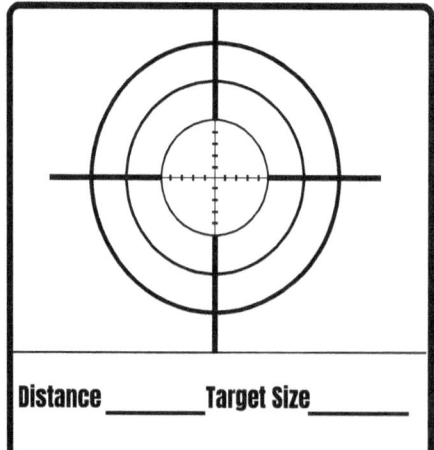

Distance _____ Target Size _____

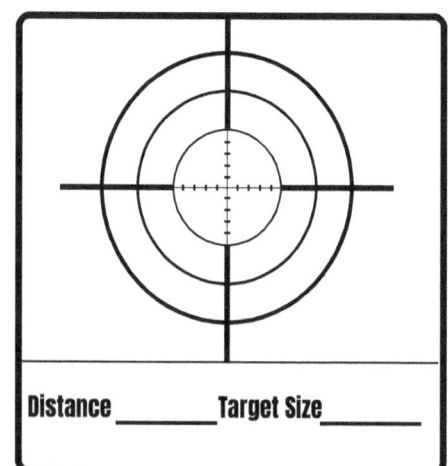

Distance _____ Target Size _____

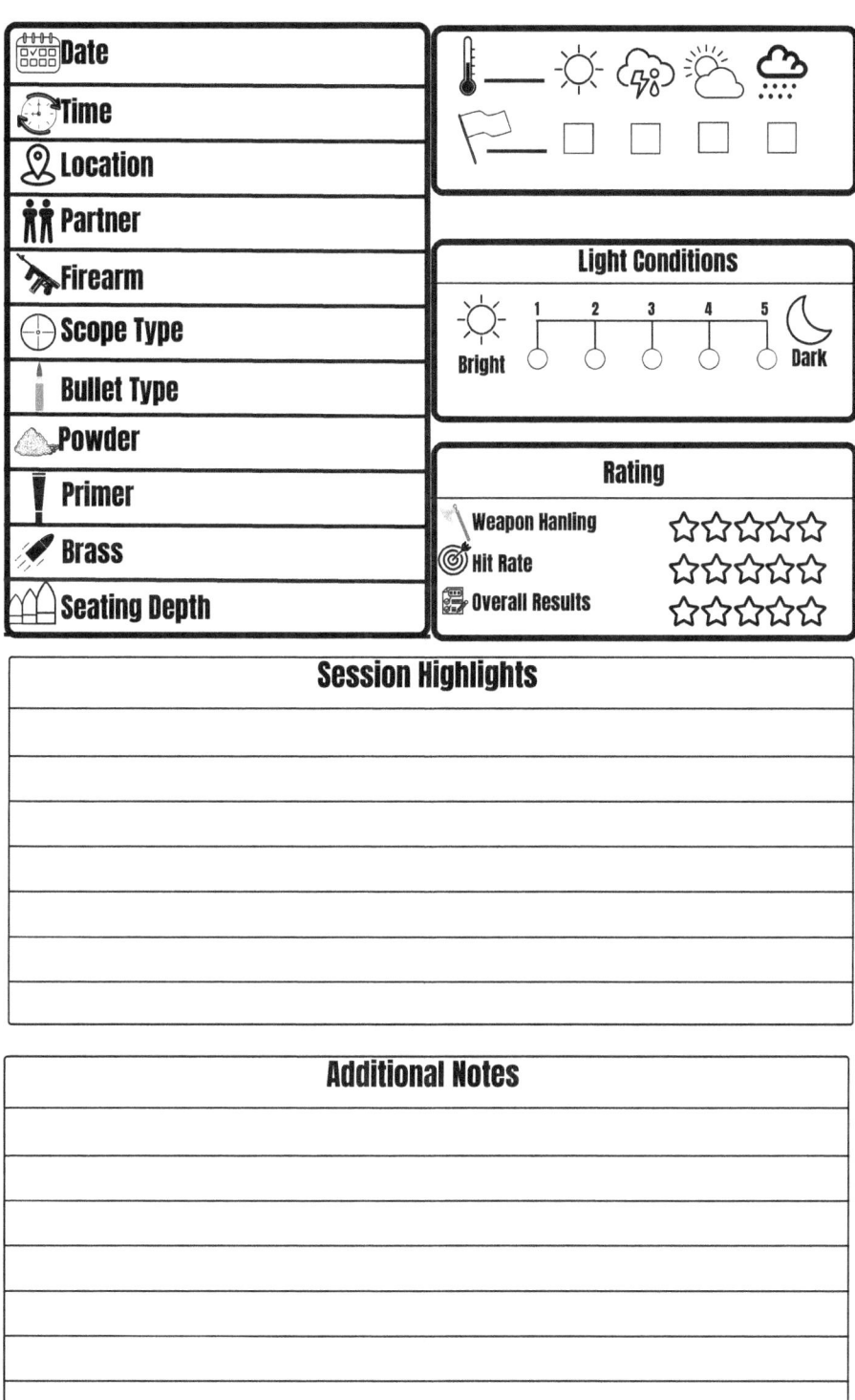

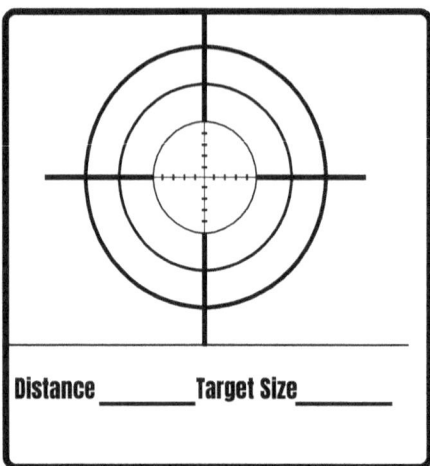
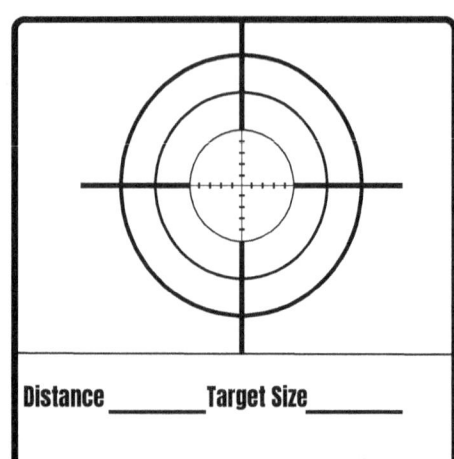
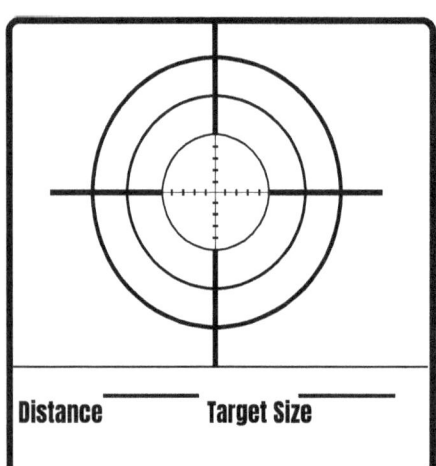
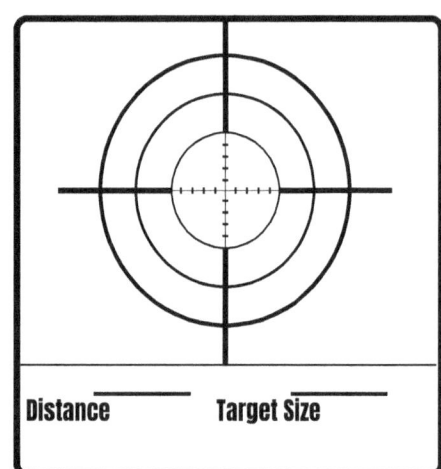
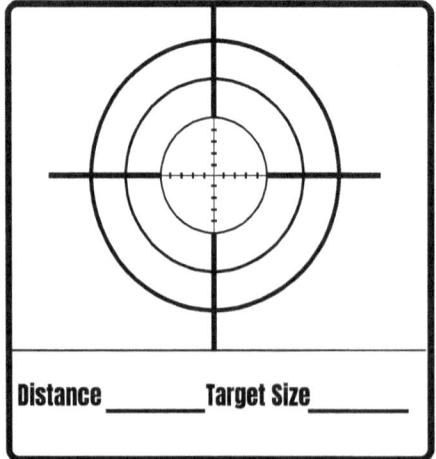
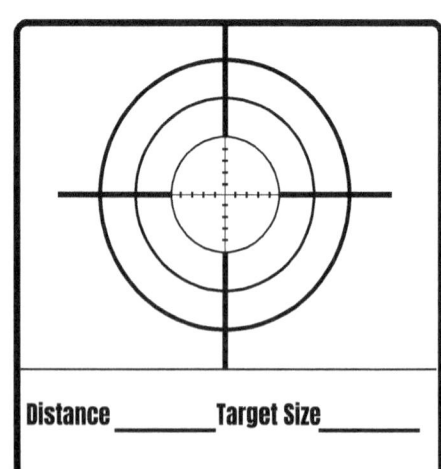

📅 Date	
⏱ Time	
📍 Location	
👥 Partner	
🔫 Firearm	
🔭 Scope Type	
🔹 Bullet Type	
Powder	
Primer	
Brass	
Seating Depth	

Weather: 🌡 ____ ☀️ ☐ ⛈ ☐ ⛅ ☐ ☁️ ☐

🚩 ____

Light Conditions

Bright ☀️ — 1 ○ — 2 ○ — 3 ○ — 4 ○ — 5 ○ 🌙 Dark

Rating

Weapon Hanling	☆☆☆☆☆
Hit Rate	☆☆☆☆☆
Overall Results	☆☆☆☆☆

Session Highlights

_____
_____
_____
_____
_____
_____
_____
_____
_____
_____

Additional Notes

_____
_____
_____
_____
_____
_____
_____
_____
_____

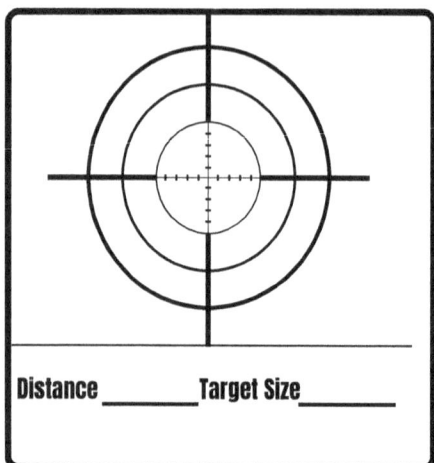

Distance _____ Target Size _____

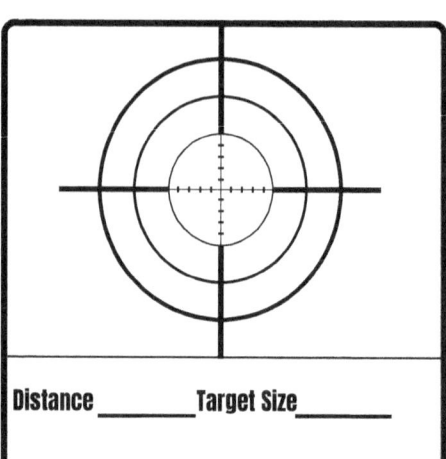

Distance _____ Target Size _____

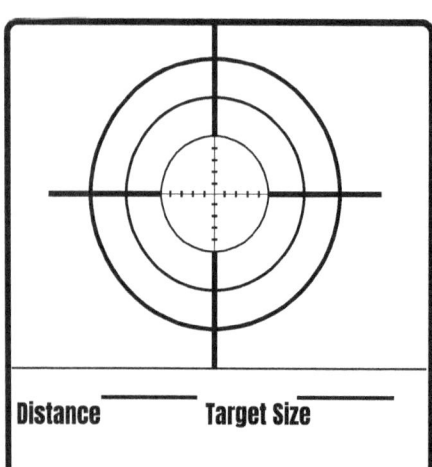

Distance _____ Target Size _____

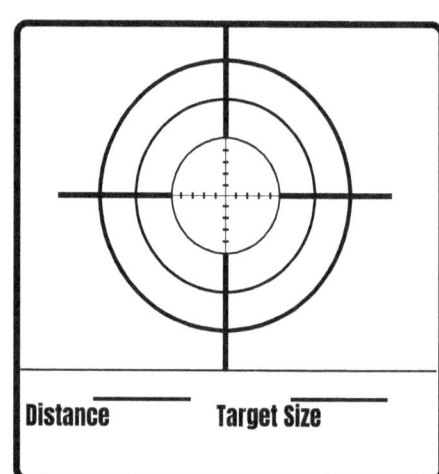

Distance _____ Target Size _____

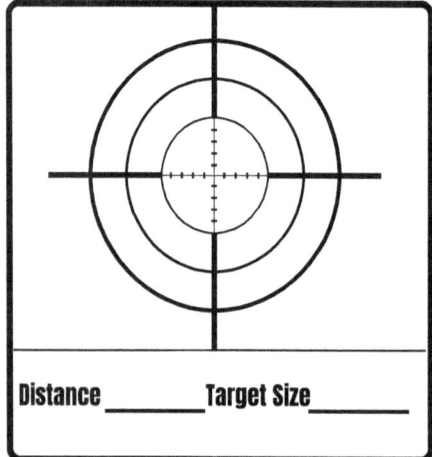

Distance _____ Target Size _____

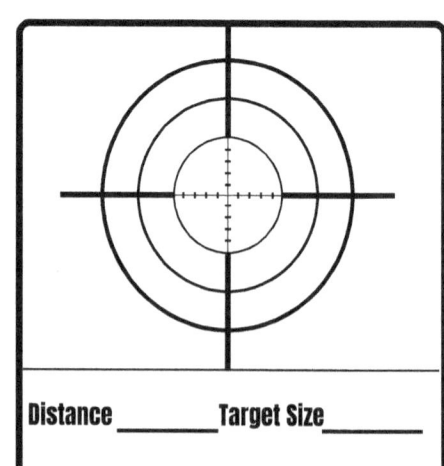

Distance _____ Target Size _____

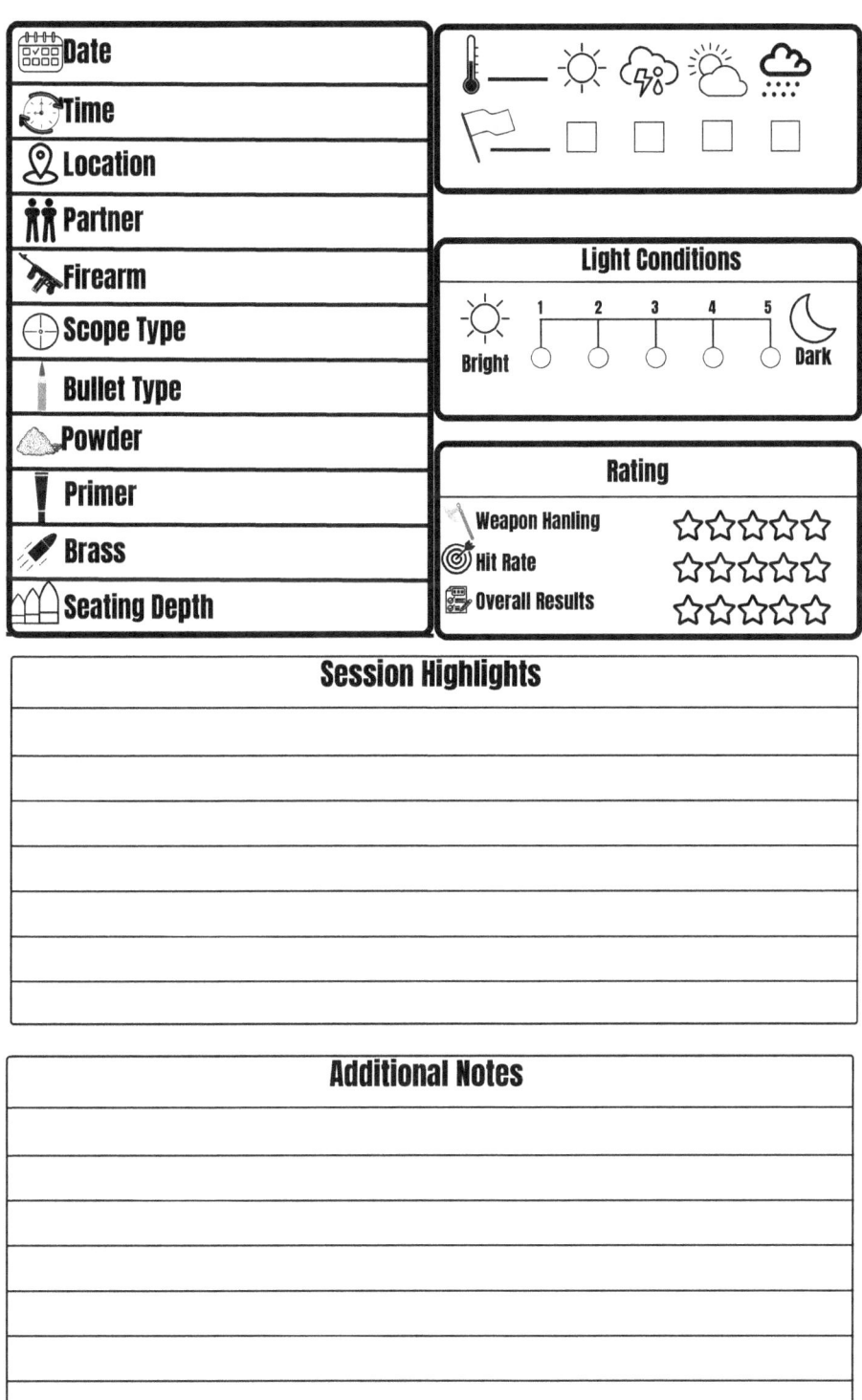

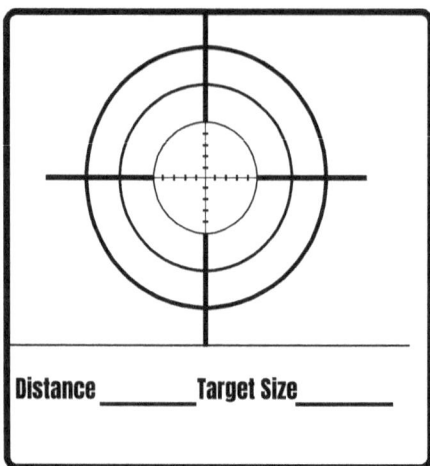
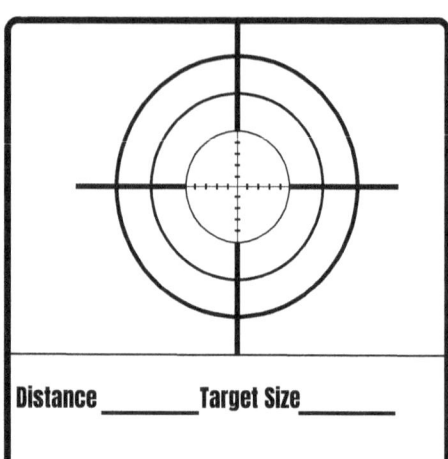
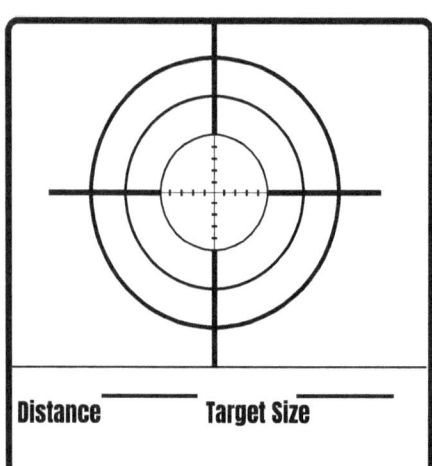
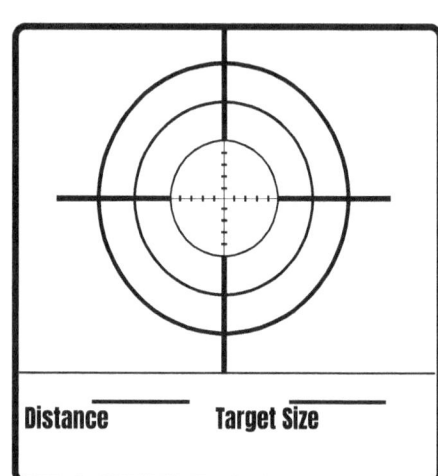
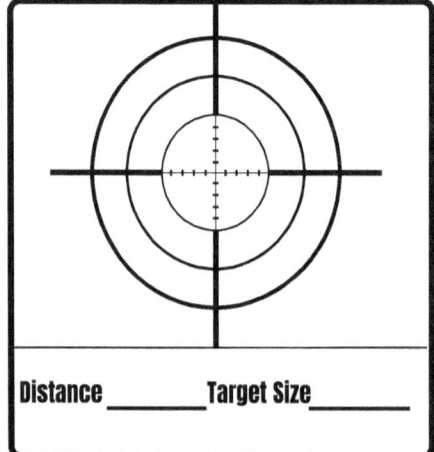
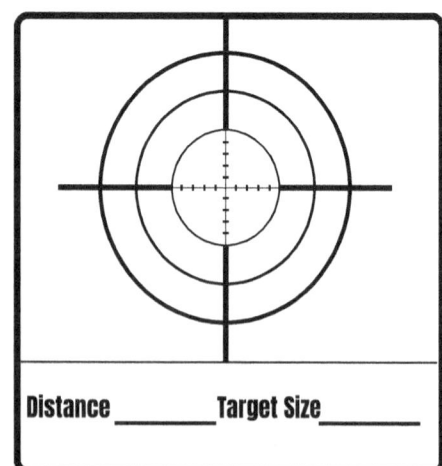

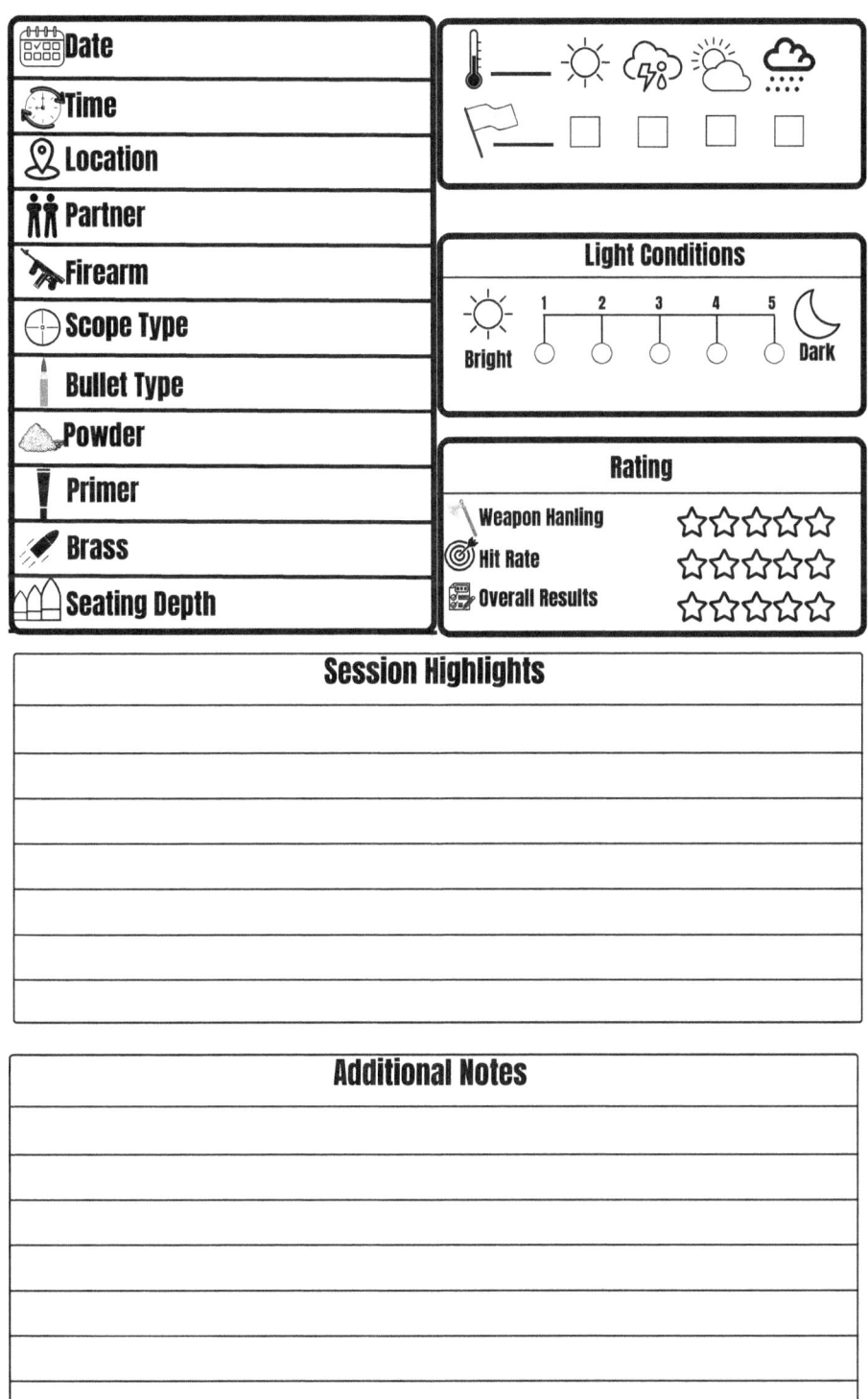

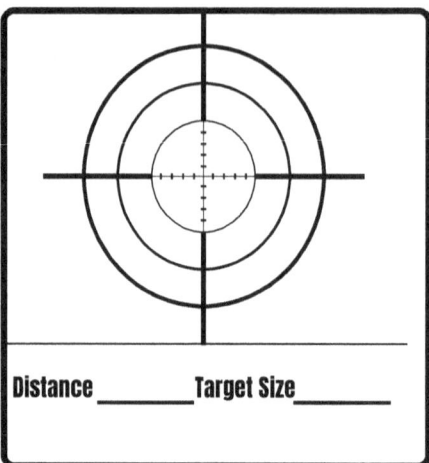
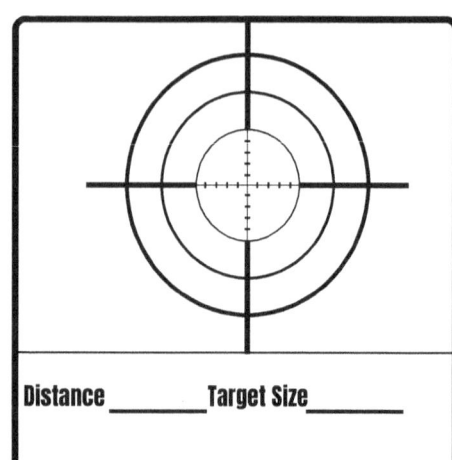
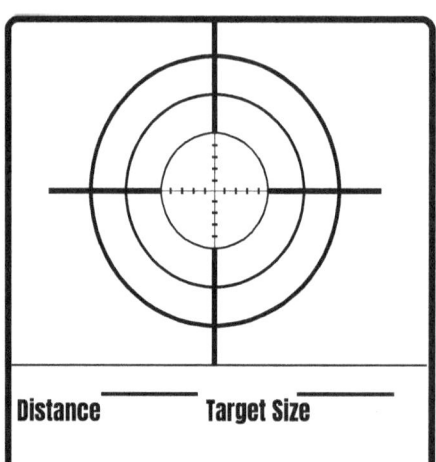
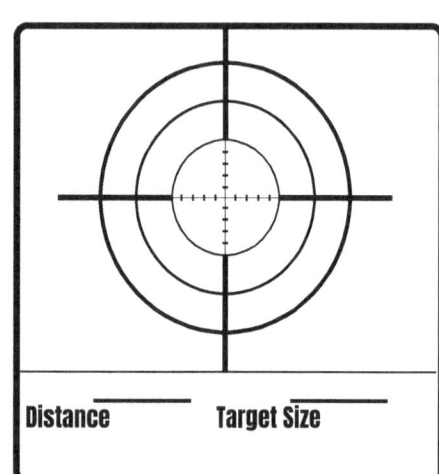
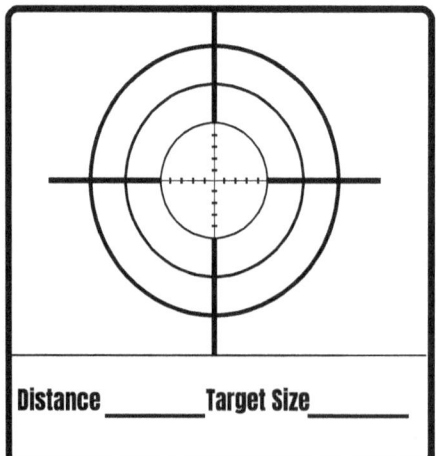
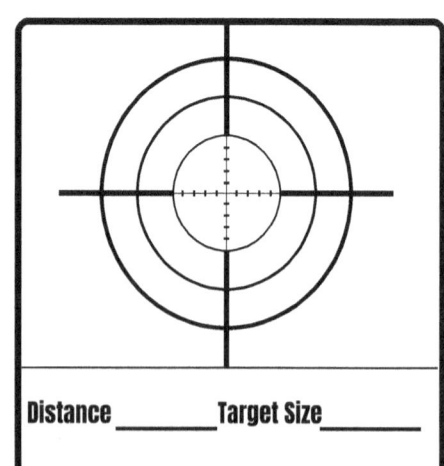

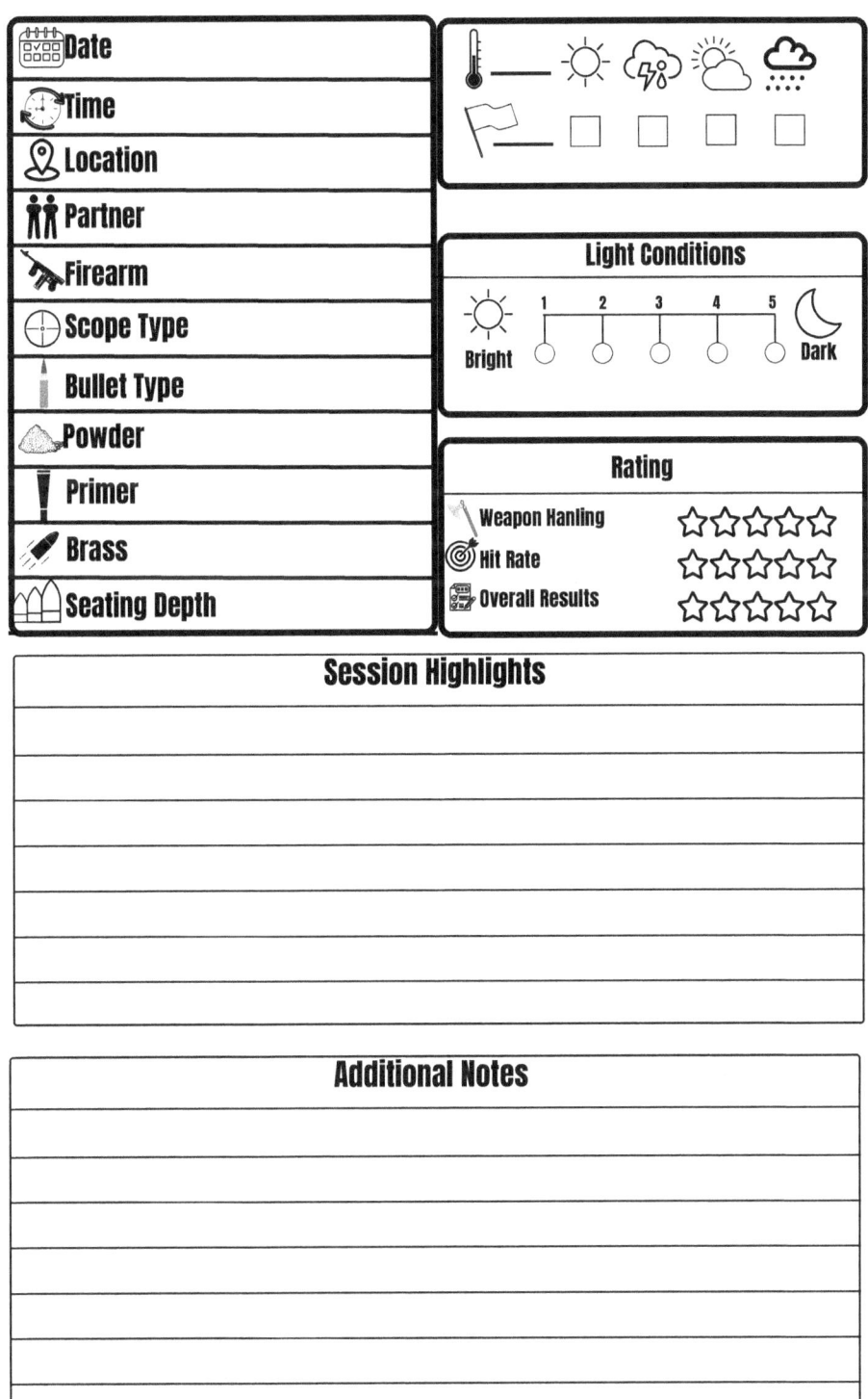

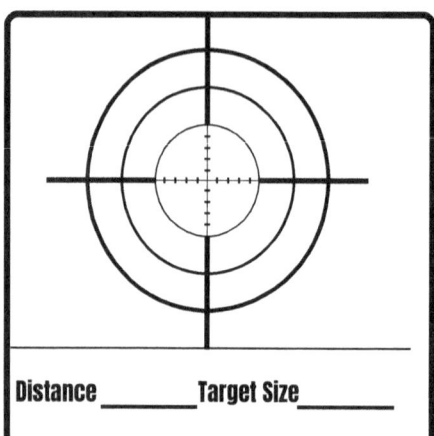

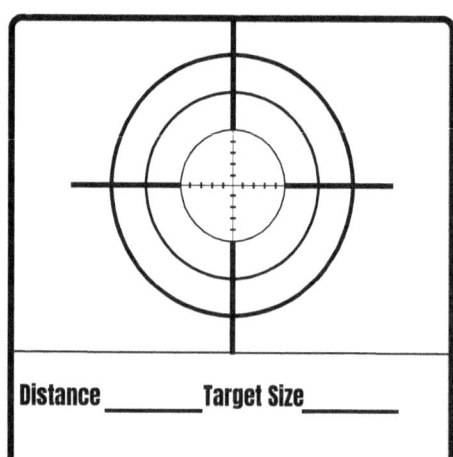

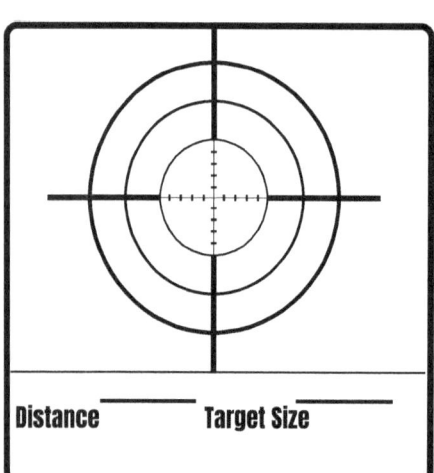

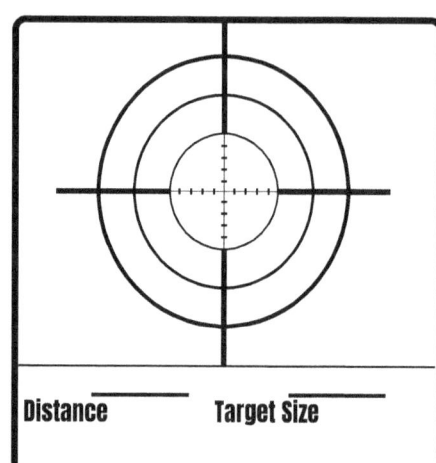

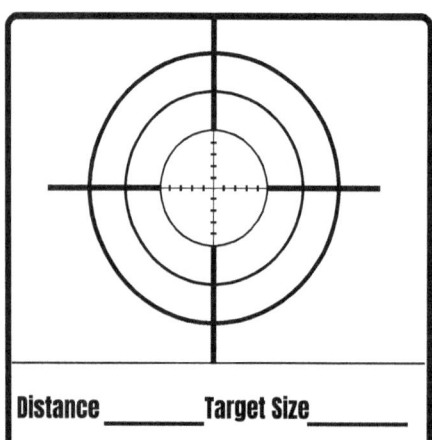

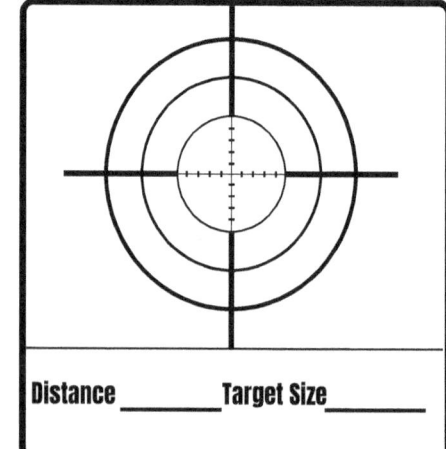

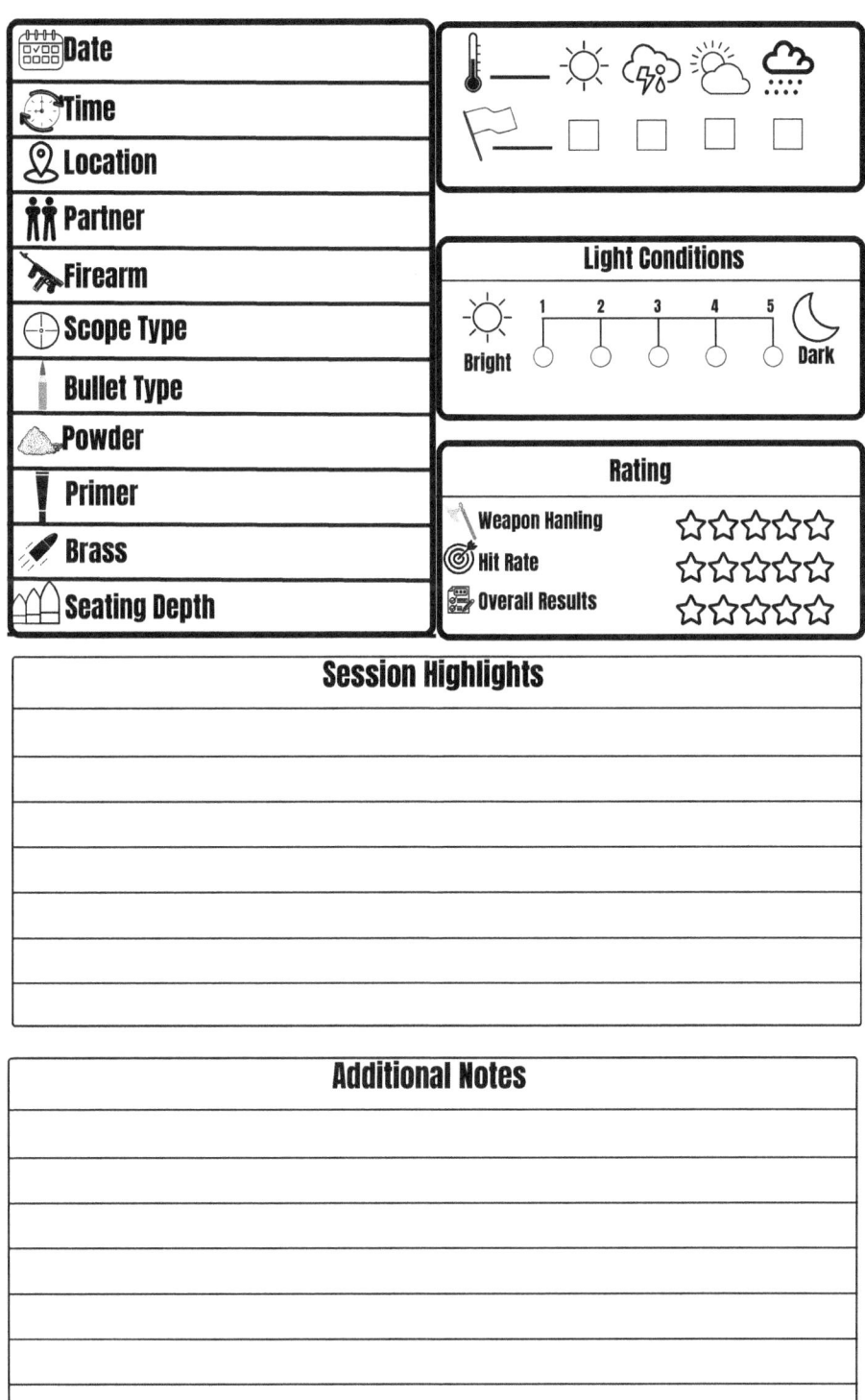

| Date |
| Time |
| Location |
| Partner |
| Firearm |
| Scope Type |
| Bullet Type |
| Powder |
| Primer |
| Brass |
| Seating Depth |

Light Conditions
Bright 1 — 2 — 3 — 4 — 5 Dark

Rating
- Weapon Hanling ☆☆☆☆☆
- Hit Rate ☆☆☆☆☆
- Overall Results ☆☆☆☆☆

Session Highlights

Additional Notes

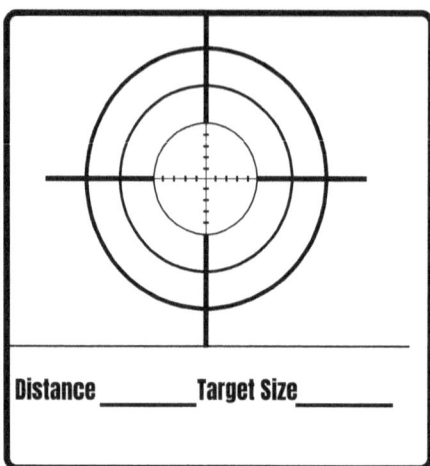
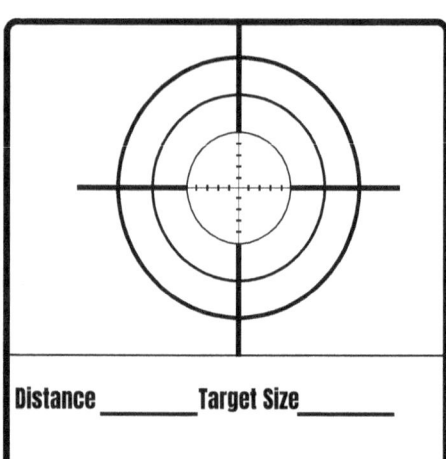
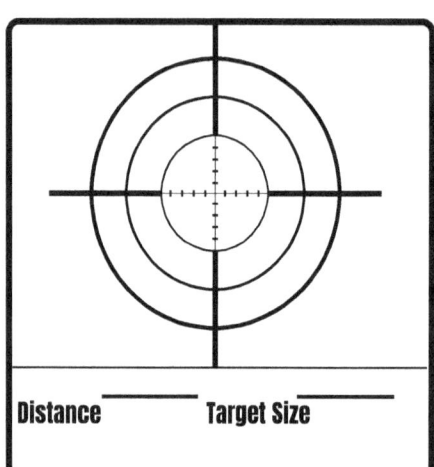
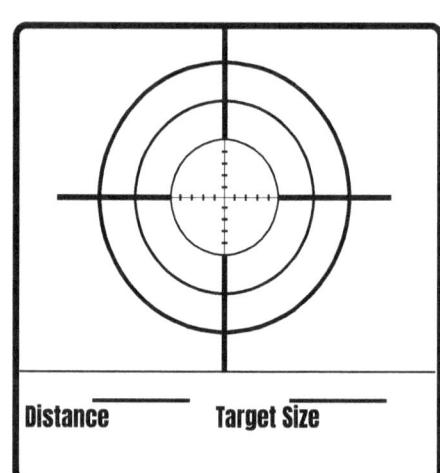
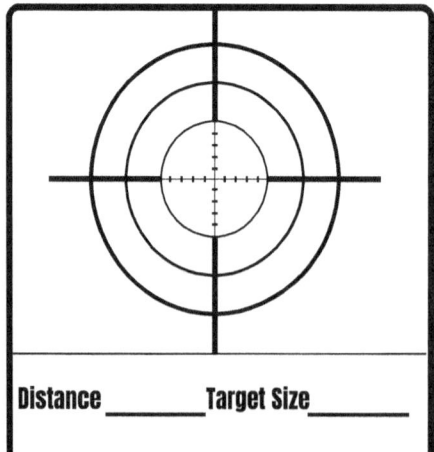
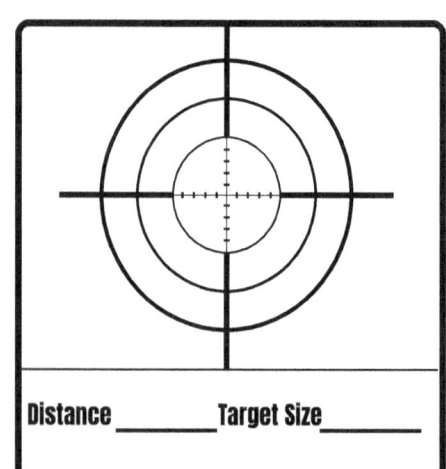

- Date
- Time
- Location
- Partner
- Firearm
- Scope Type
- Bullet Type
- Powder
- Primer
- Brass
- Seating Depth

Light Conditions

Bright 1 2 3 4 5 Dark

Rating

- Weapon Hanling ☆☆☆☆☆
- Hit Rate ☆☆☆☆☆
- Overall Results ☆☆☆☆☆

Session Highlights

Additional Notes

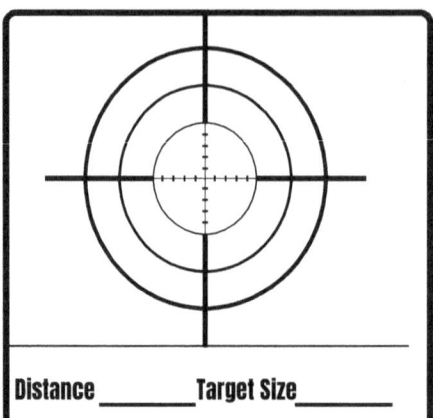

Distance _____ Target Size _____

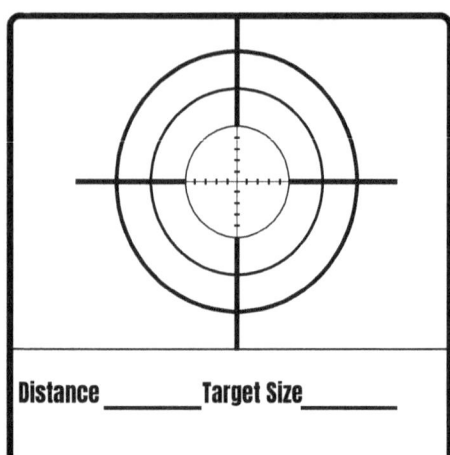

Distance _____ Target Size _____

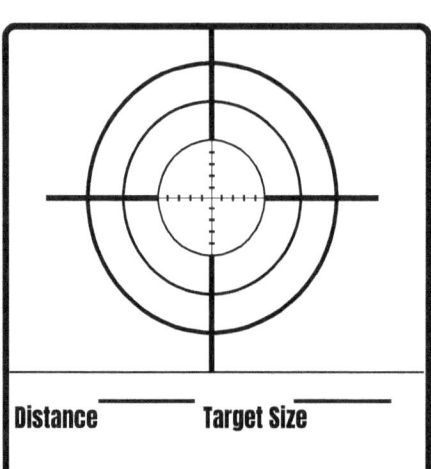

Distance _____ Target Size _____

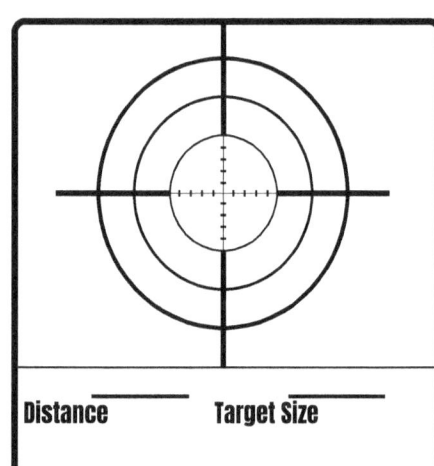

Distance _____ Target Size _____

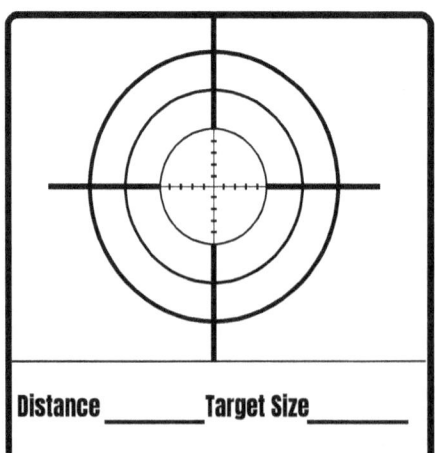

Distance _____ Target Size _____

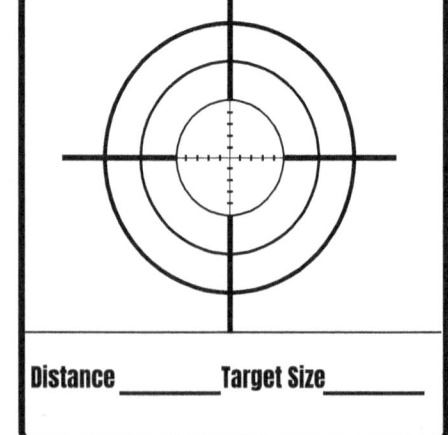

Distance _____ Target Size _____

Date	
Time	
Location	
Partner	
Firearm	
Scope Type	
Bullet Type	
Powder	
Primer	
Brass	
Seating Depth	

Light Conditions

Bright 1 — 2 — 3 — 4 — 5 Dark

Rating

Weapon Hanling	☆☆☆☆☆
Hit Rate	☆☆☆☆☆
Overall Results	☆☆☆☆☆

Session Highlights

Additional Notes

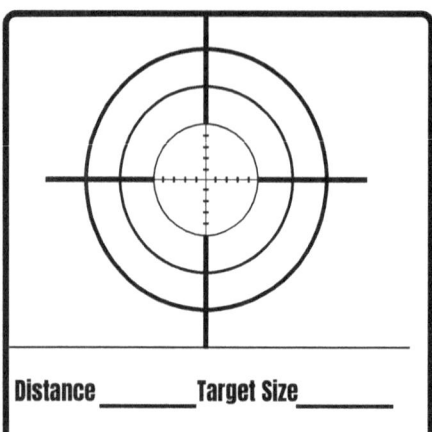

Distance _____ Target Size _____

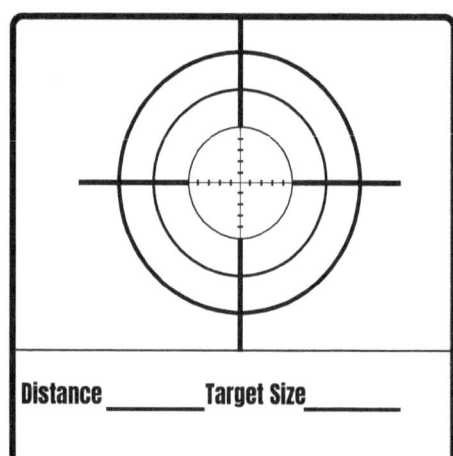

Distance _____ Target Size _____

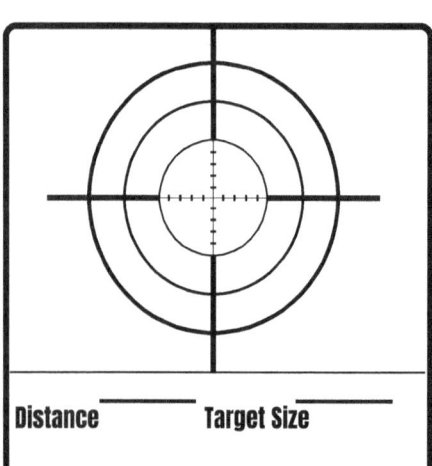

Distance _____ Target Size _____

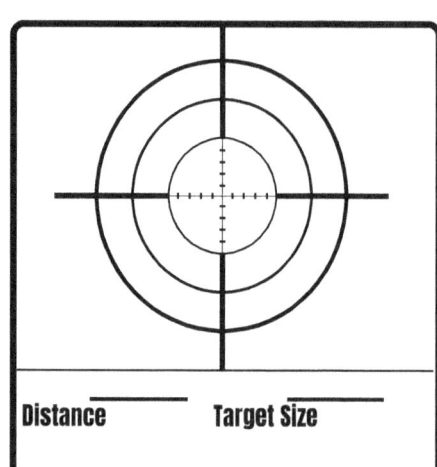

Distance _____ Target Size _____

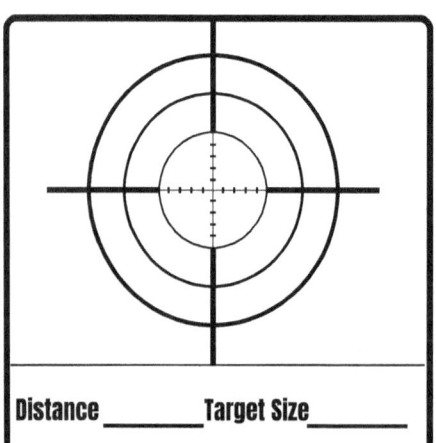

Distance _____ Target Size _____

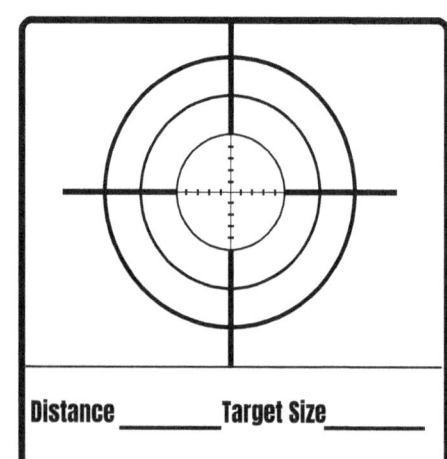

Distance _____ Target Size _____

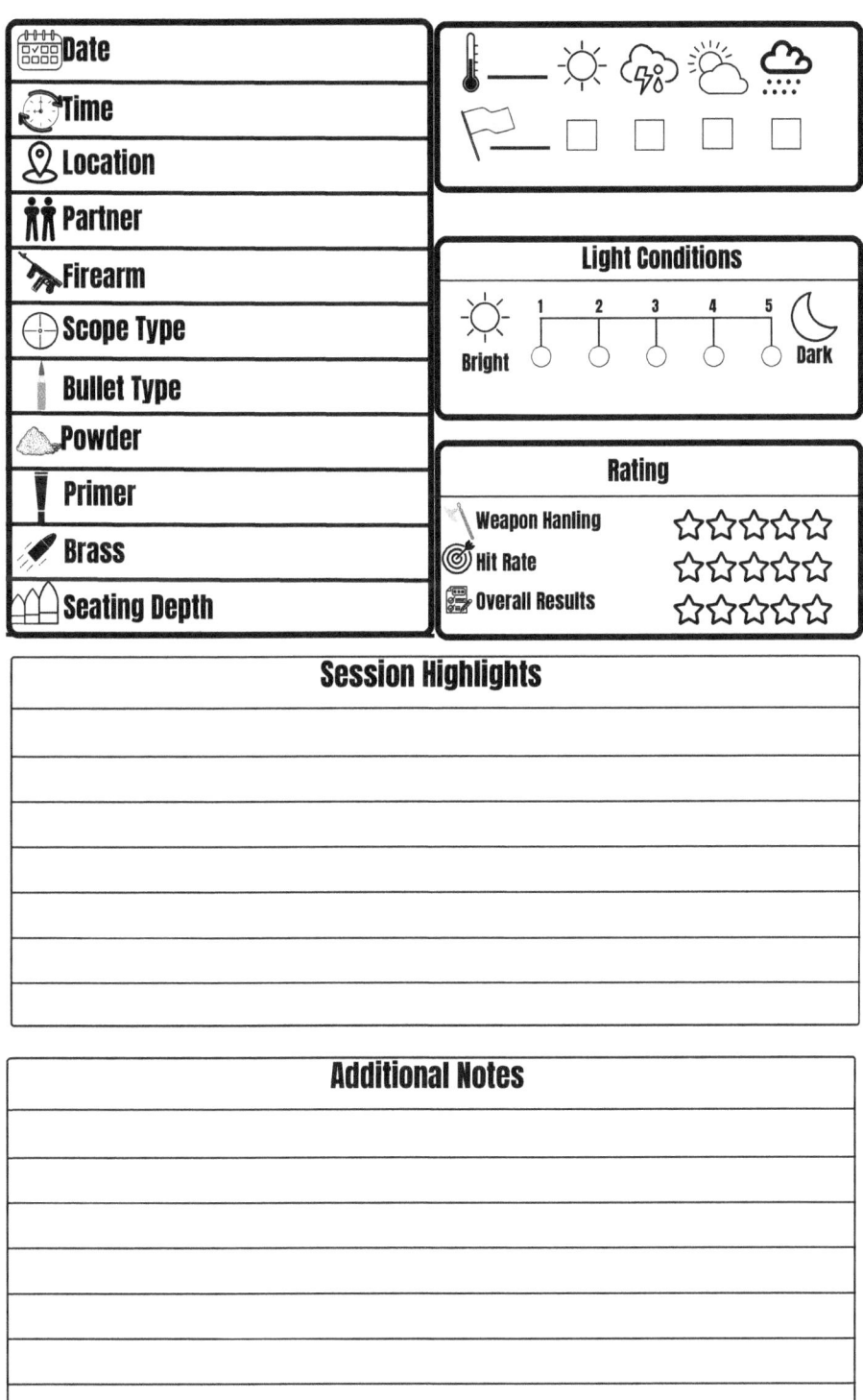

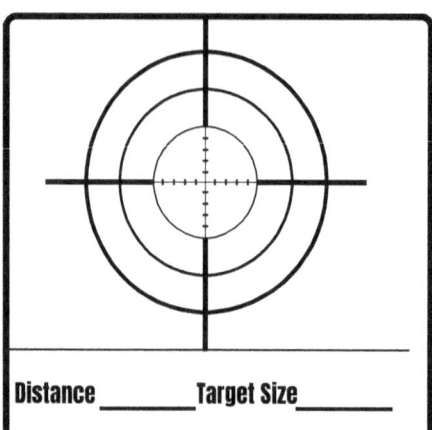
Distance _____ Target Size _____

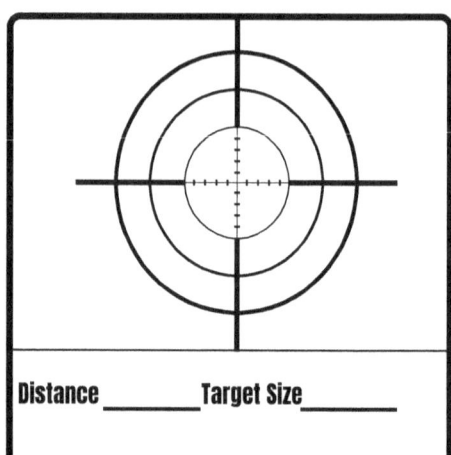
Distance _____ Target Size _____

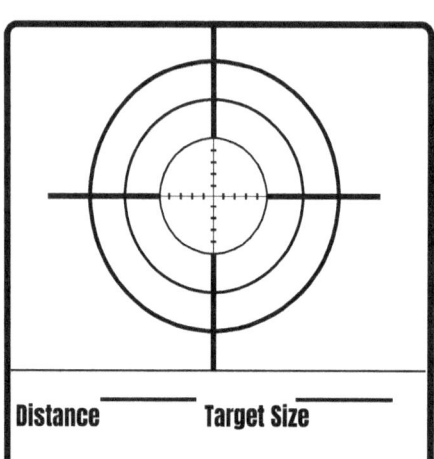
Distance _____ Target Size _____

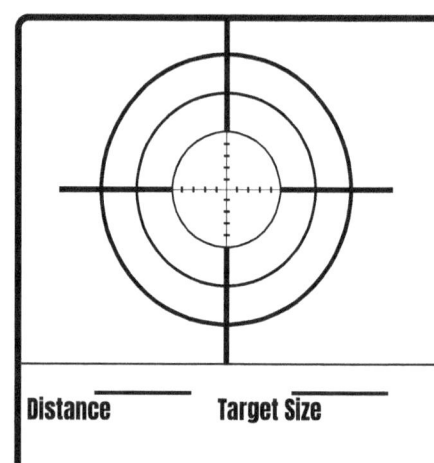
Distance _____ Target Size _____

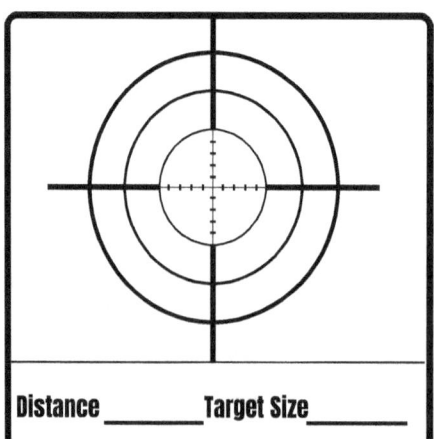
Distance _____ Target Size _____

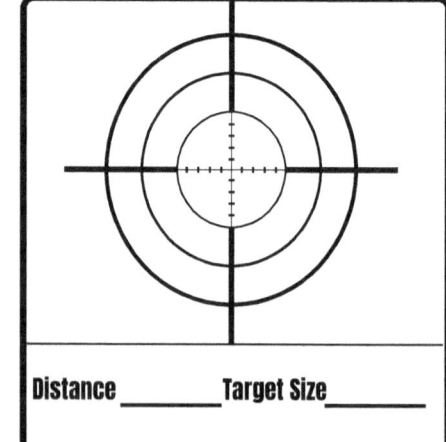
Distance _____ Target Size _____

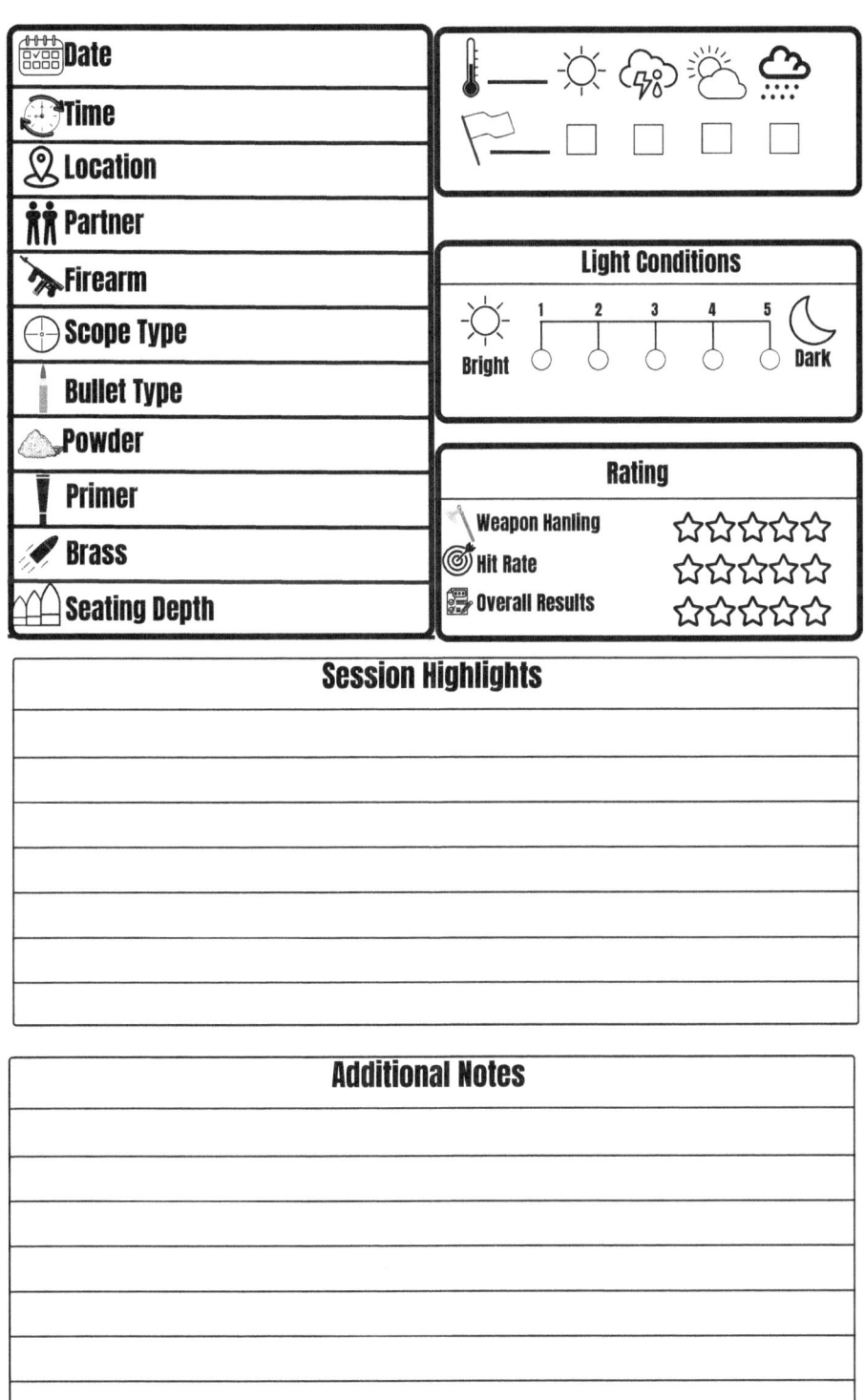

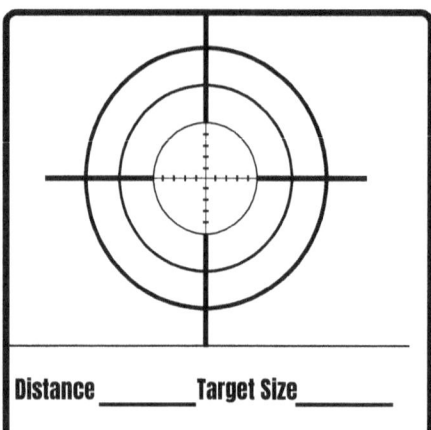
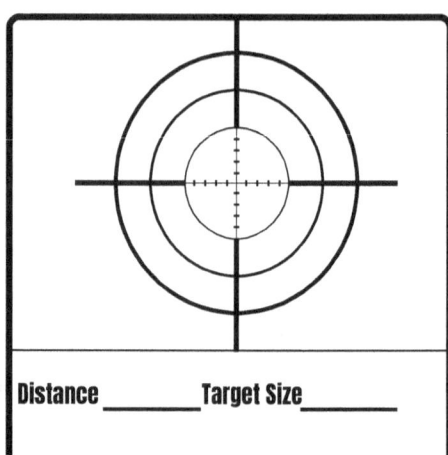
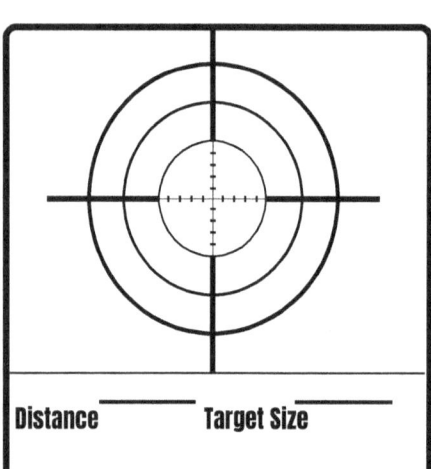
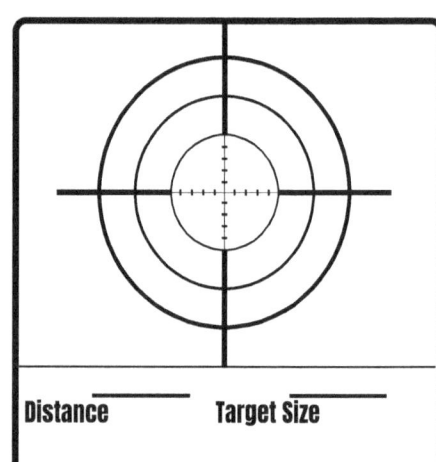
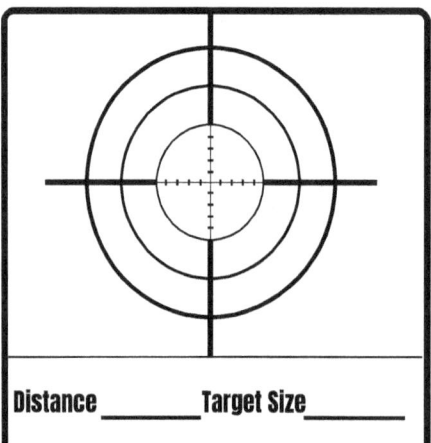
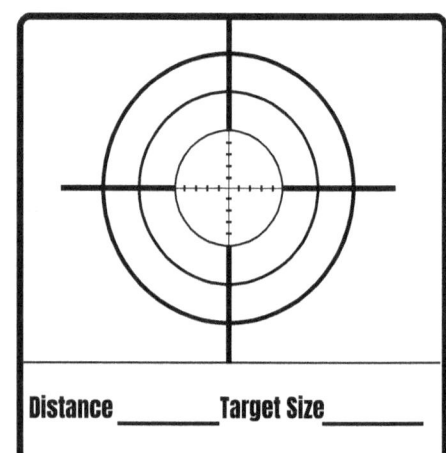

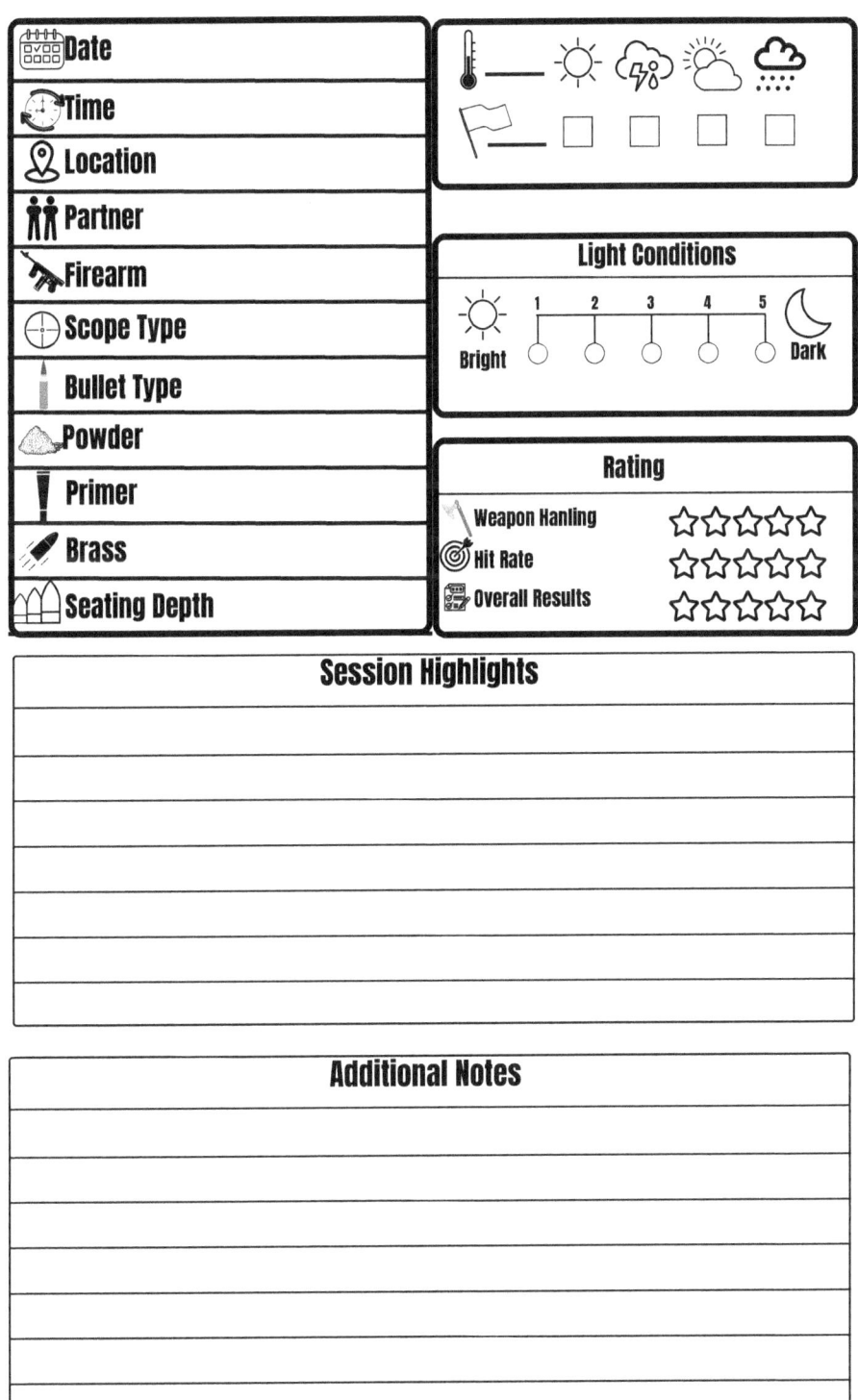

Date	
Time	
Location	
Partner	
Firearm	
Scope Type	
Bullet Type	
Powder	
Primer	
Brass	
Seating Depth	

Light Conditions

Bright 1 2 3 4 5 Dark

Rating

- Weapon Hanling ☆☆☆☆☆
- Hit Rate ☆☆☆☆☆
- Overall Results ☆☆☆☆☆

Session Highlights

Additional Notes

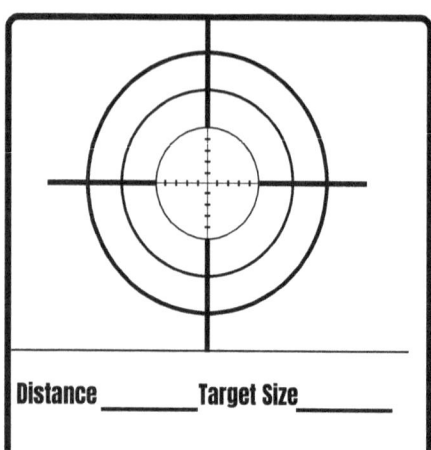
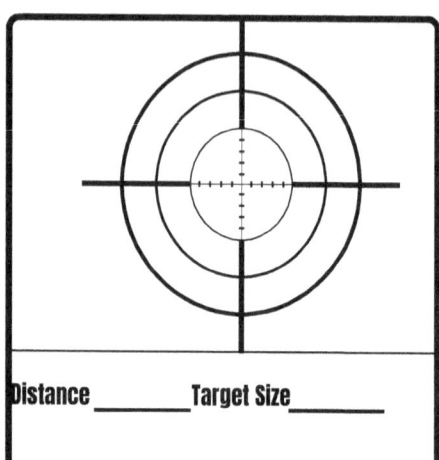
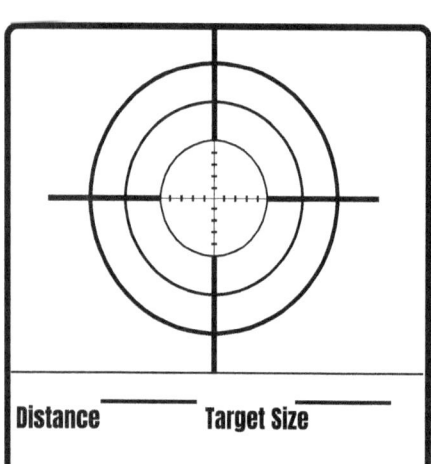
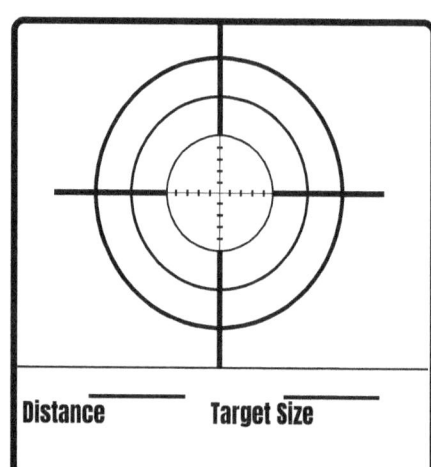
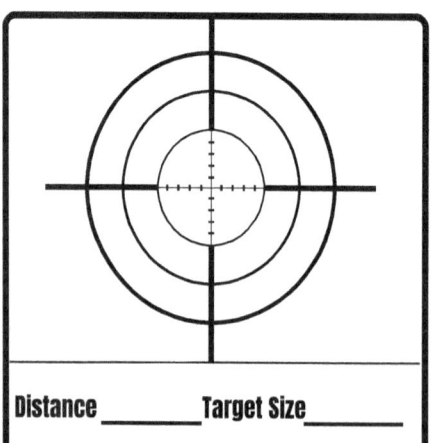
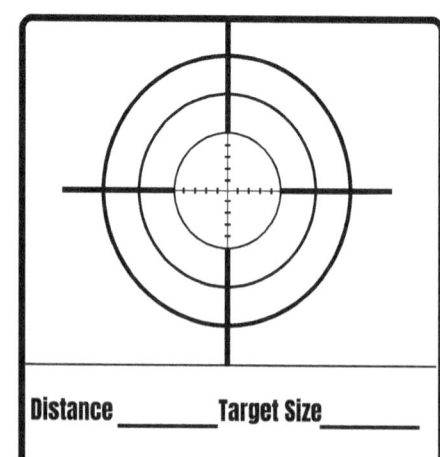

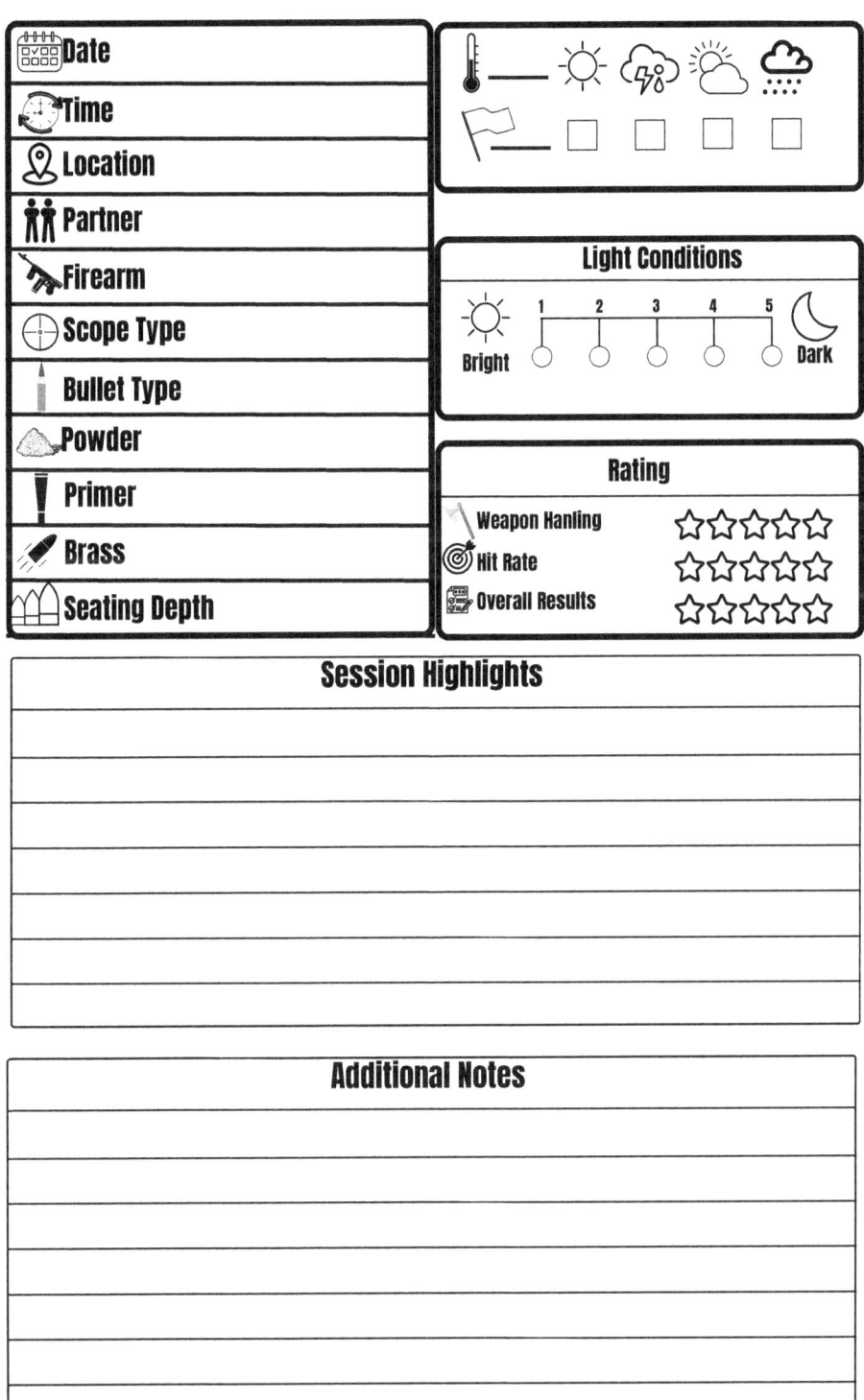

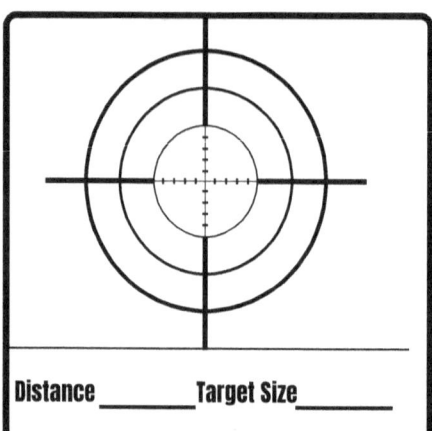

Distance _____Target Size_____

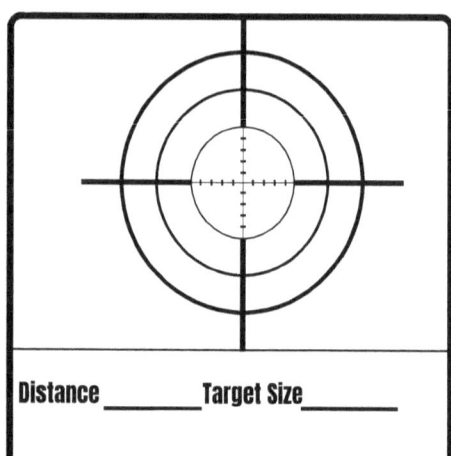

Distance _____Target Size_____

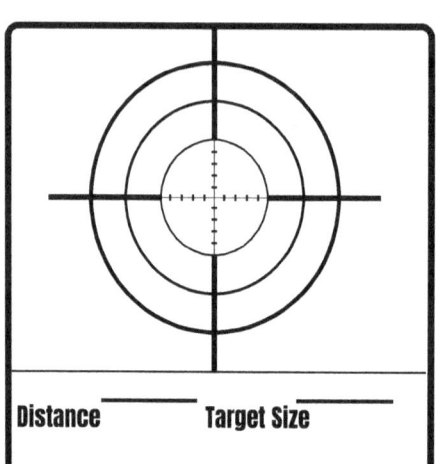

Distance _____Target Size_____

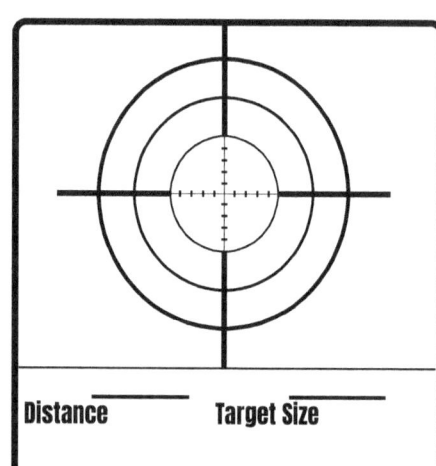

Distance _____Target Size_____

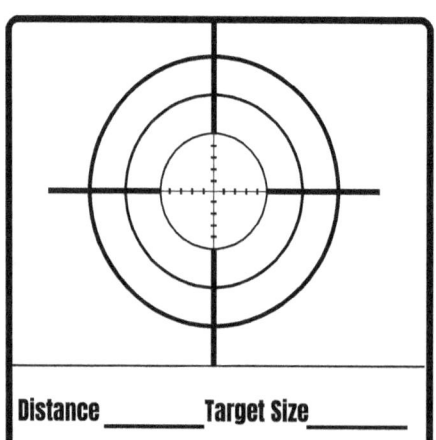

Distance _____Target Size_____

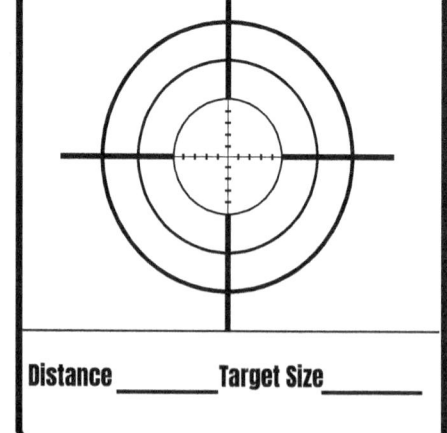

Distance _____Target Size_____

📅 Date	
⏱ Time	
📍 Location	
👥 Partner	
🔫 Firearm	
🔭 Scope Type	
Bullet Type	
Powder	
Primer	
Brass	
Seating Depth	

Light Conditions

Bright 1 2 3 4 5 Dark

Rating

- Weapon Hanling ☆☆☆☆☆
- Hit Rate ☆☆☆☆☆
- Overall Results ☆☆☆☆☆

Session Highlights

Additional Notes

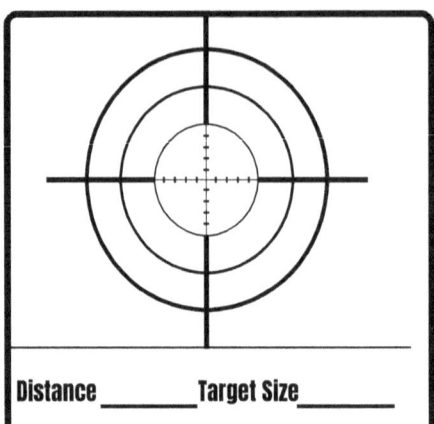
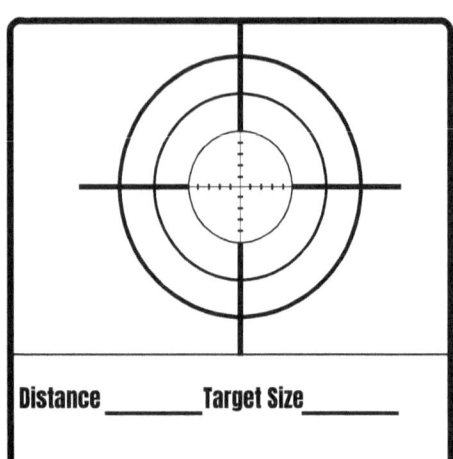
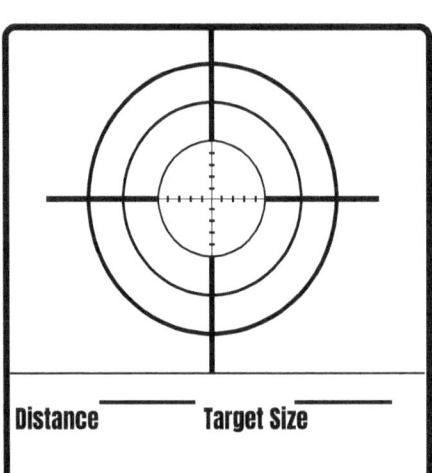
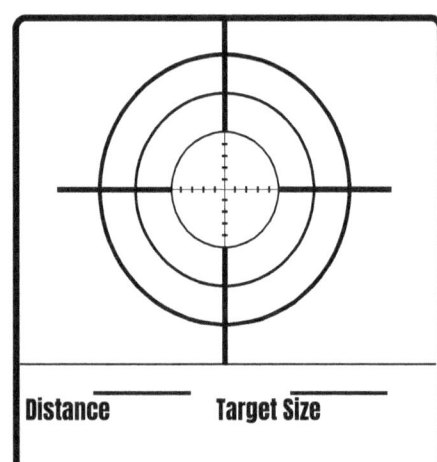
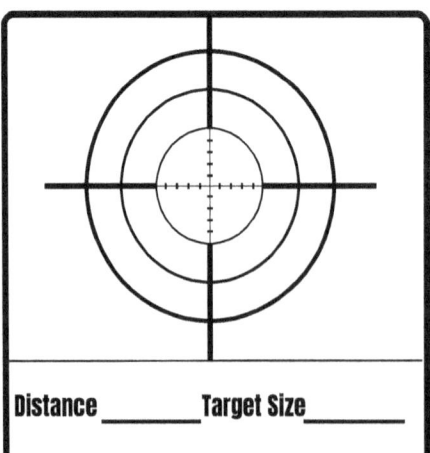
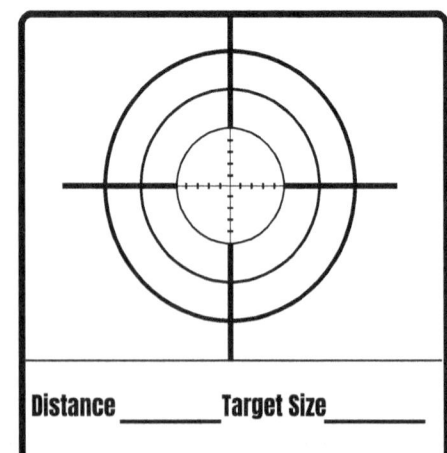

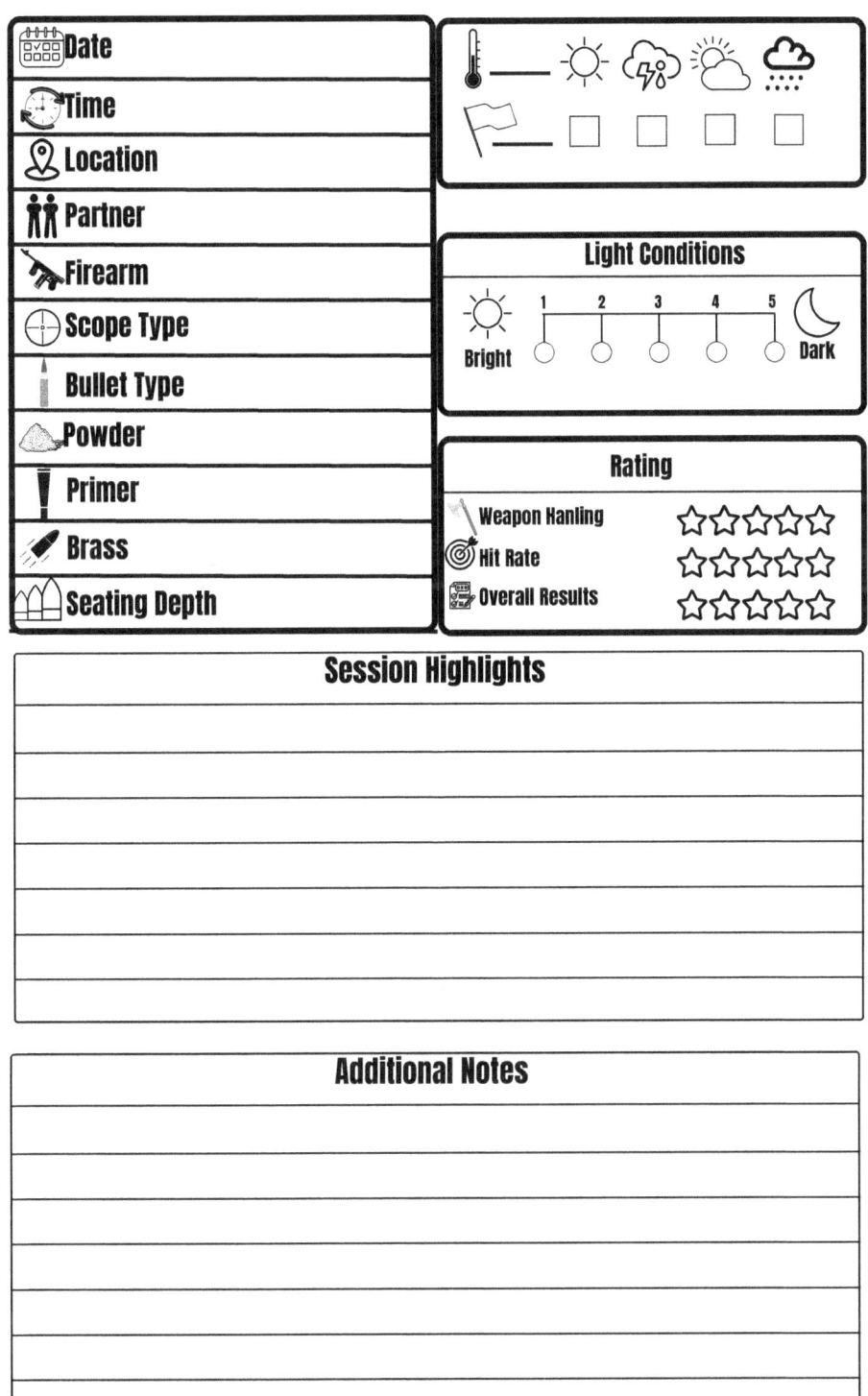

📅 Date	
⏱ Time	
📍 Location	
👥 Partner	
🔫 Firearm	
⊕ Scope Type	
🔋 Bullet Type	
🌀 Powder	
❗ Primer	
🚀 Brass	
🔺 Seating Depth	

Light Conditions

Bright 1 — 2 — 3 — 4 — 5 Dark

Rating

- Weapon Hanling ☆☆☆☆☆
- Hit Rate ☆☆☆☆☆
- Overall Results ☆☆☆☆☆

Session Highlights

Additional Notes

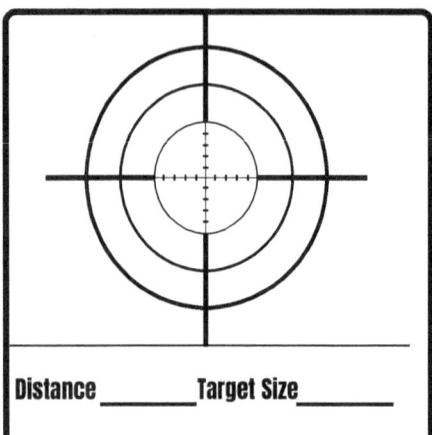
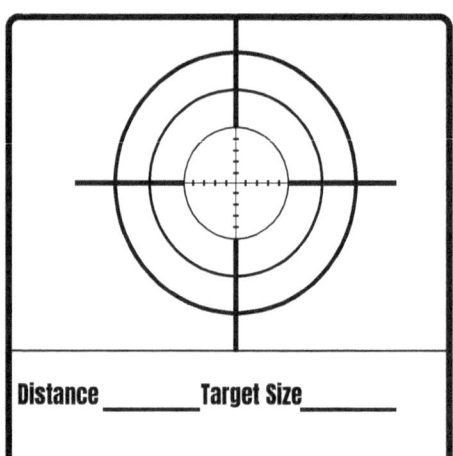
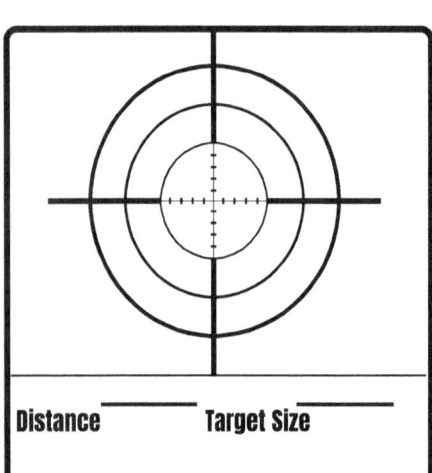
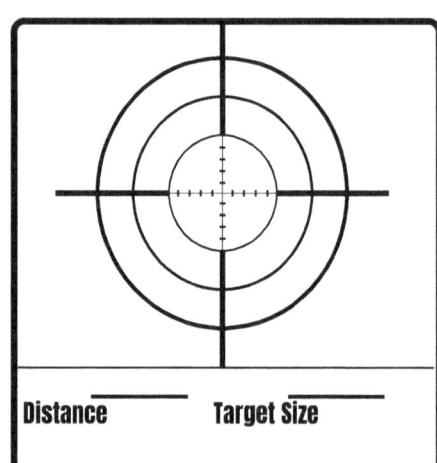
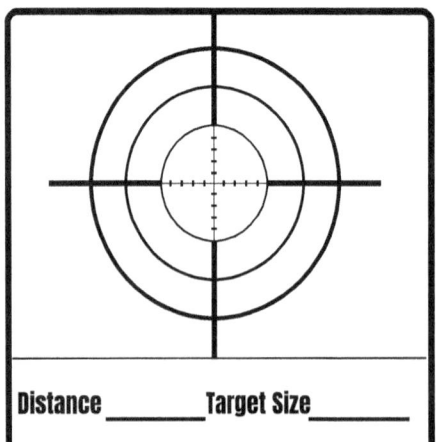
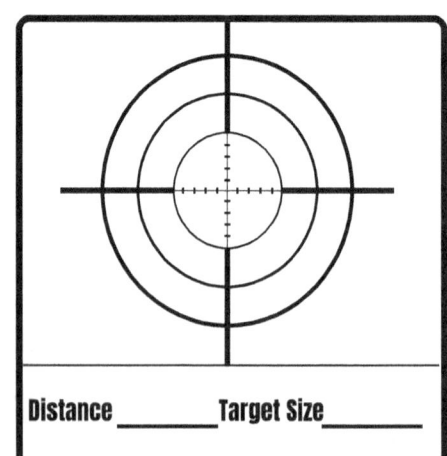

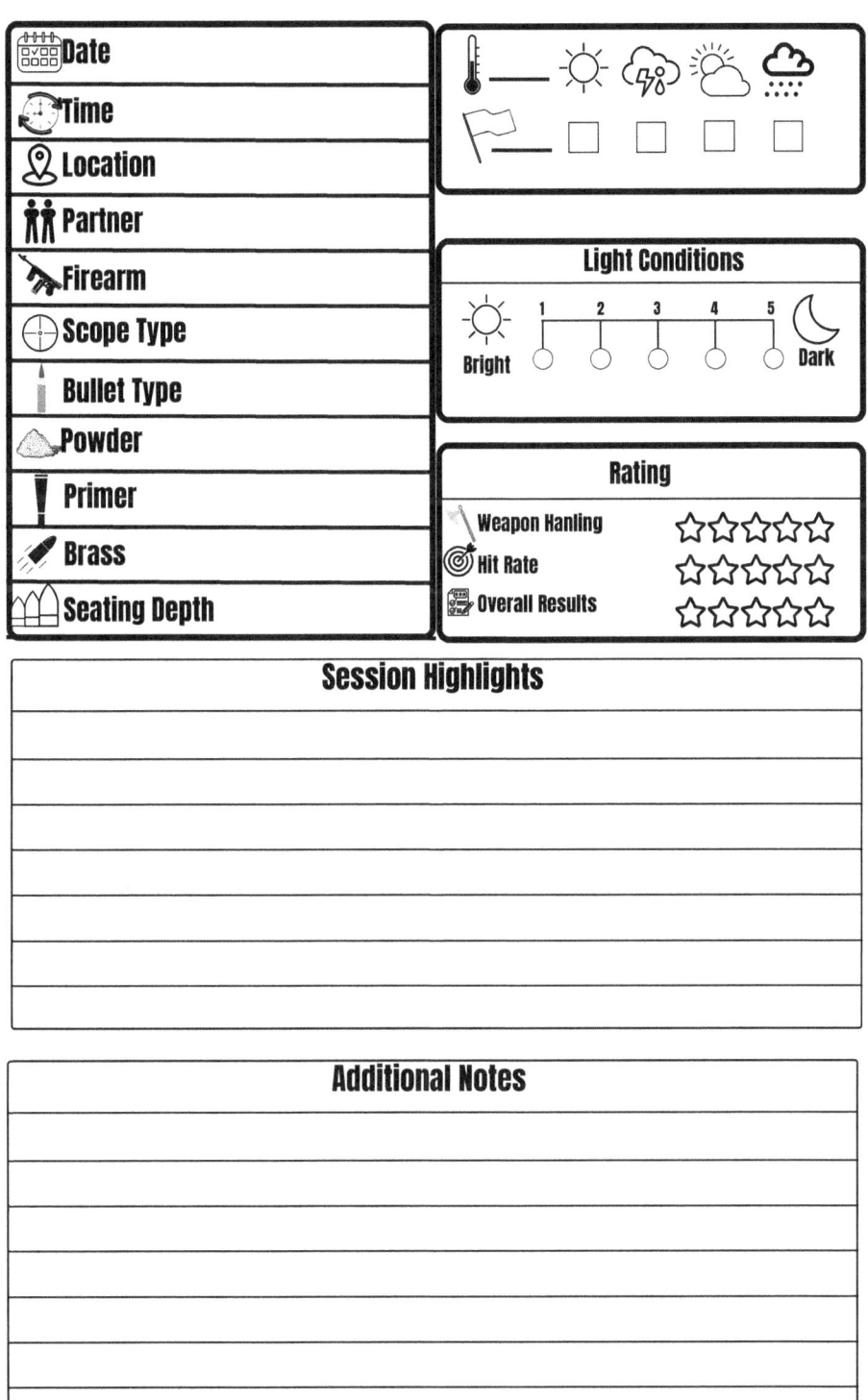

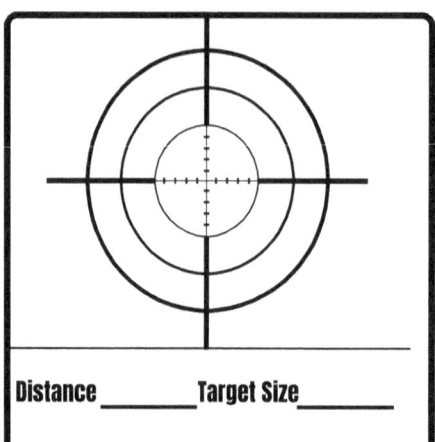
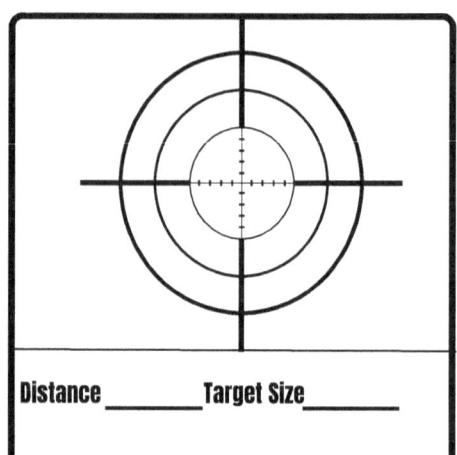
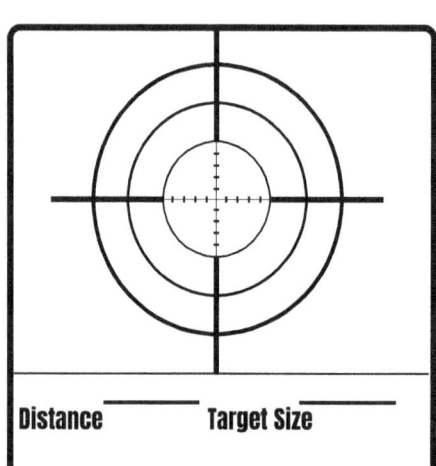
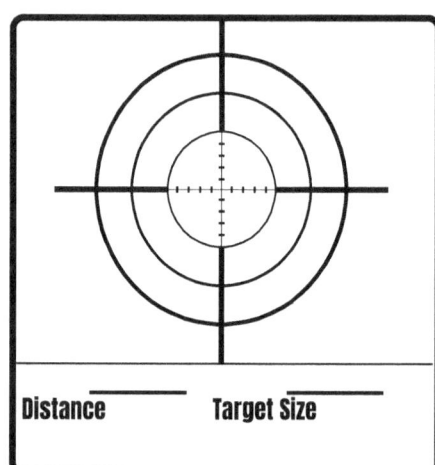
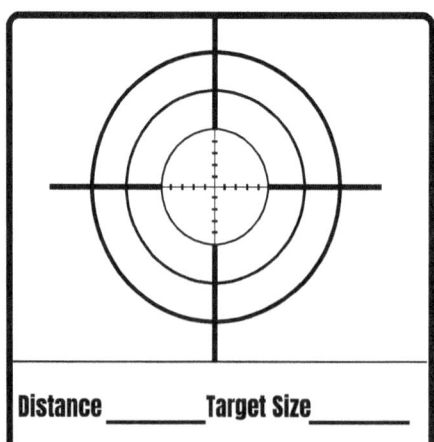
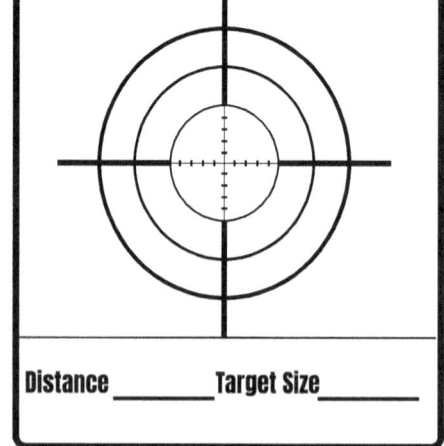

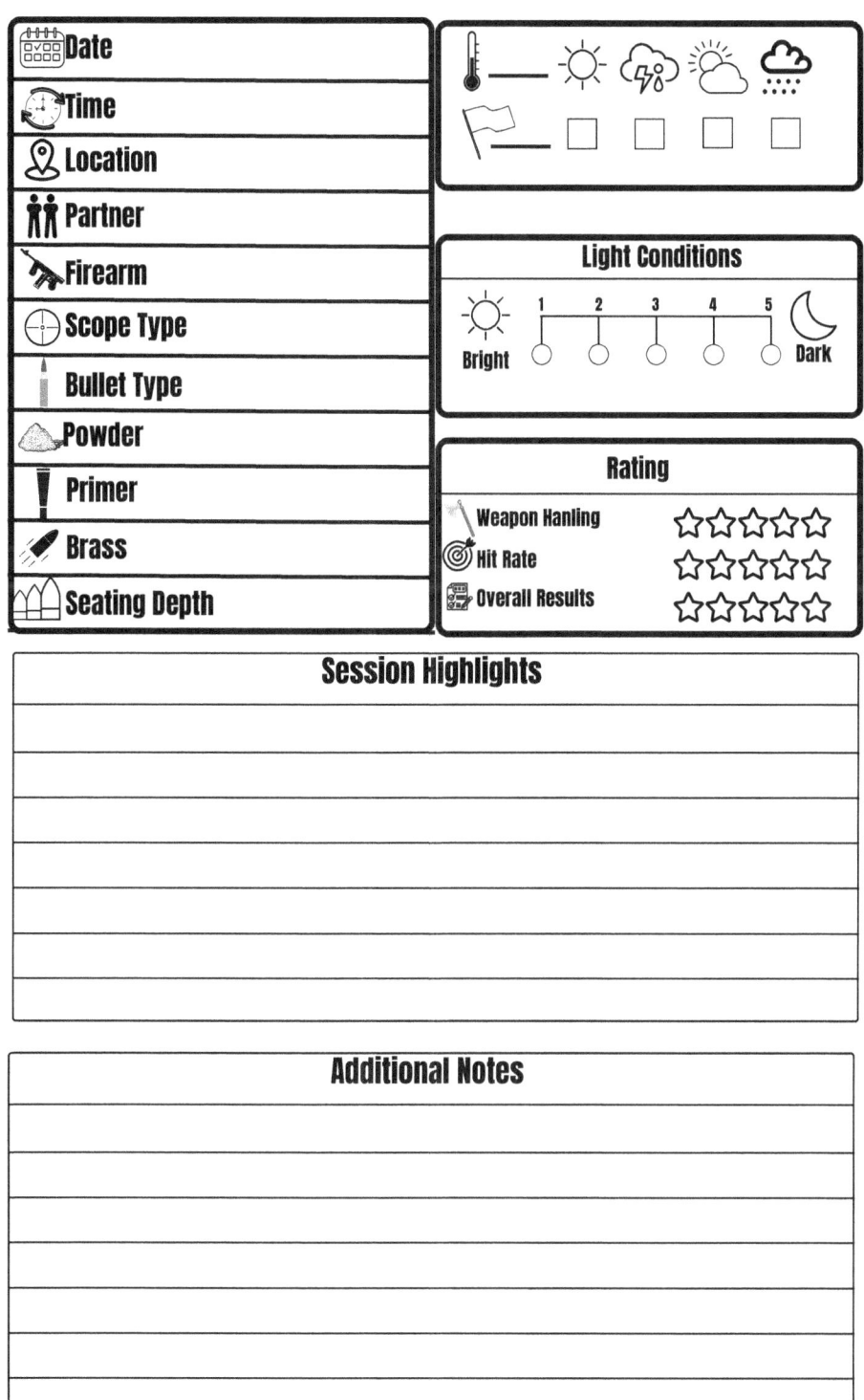

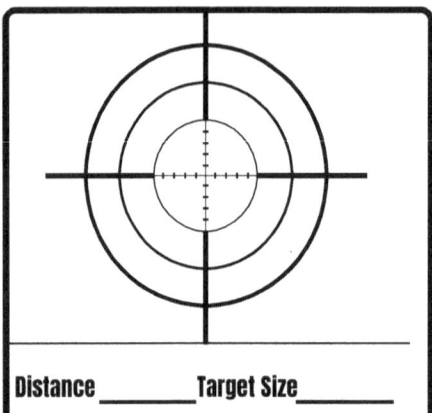

Distance _____ Target Size _____

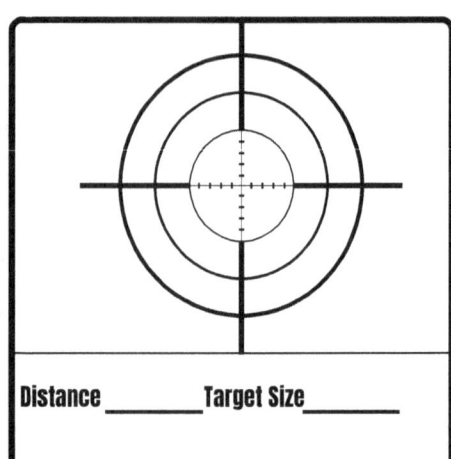

Distance _____ Target Size _____

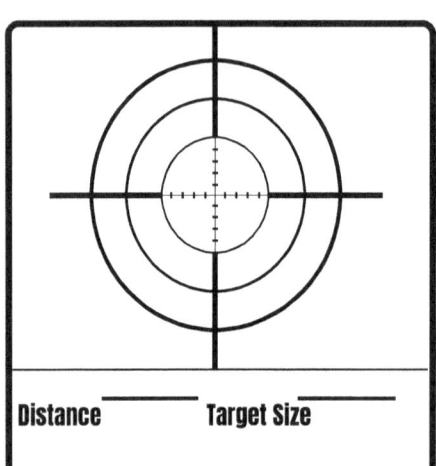

Distance _____ Target Size _____

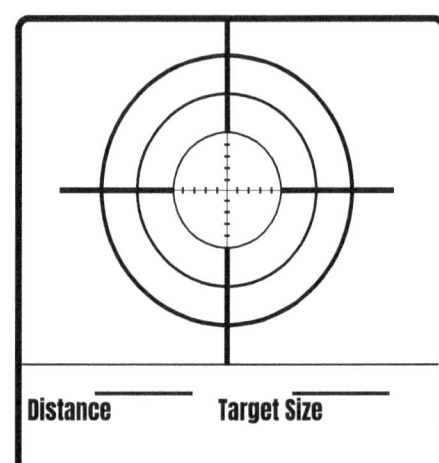

Distance _____ Target Size _____

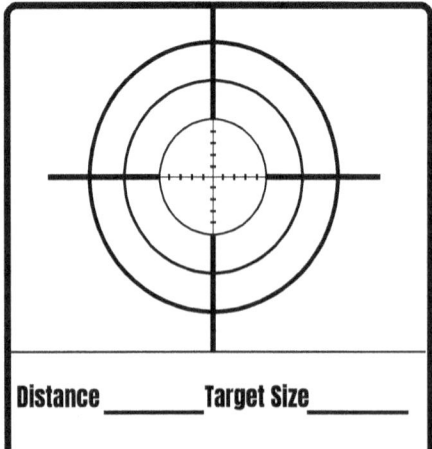

Distance _____ Target Size _____

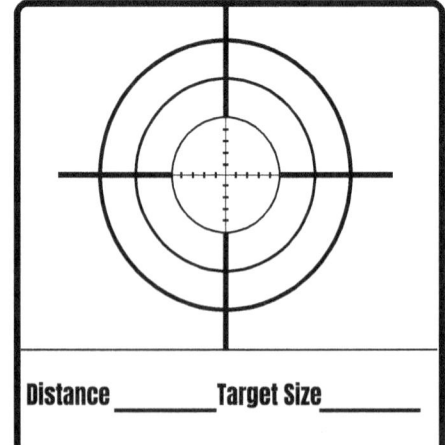

Distance _____ Target Size _____

📅 Date	
⏱ Time	
📍 Location	
👥 Partner	
🔫 Firearm	
🔭 Scope Type	
🔋 Bullet Type	
Powder	
Primer	
Brass	
Seating Depth	

Light Conditions

Bright ☀ 1 — 2 — 3 — 4 — 5 ☾ Dark

Rating

Weapon Hanling	☆☆☆☆☆
Hit Rate	☆☆☆☆☆
Overall Results	☆☆☆☆☆

Session Highlights

Additional Notes

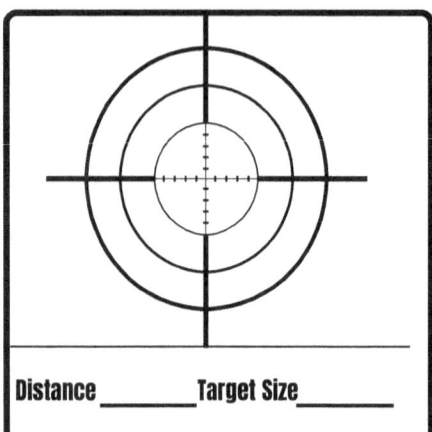
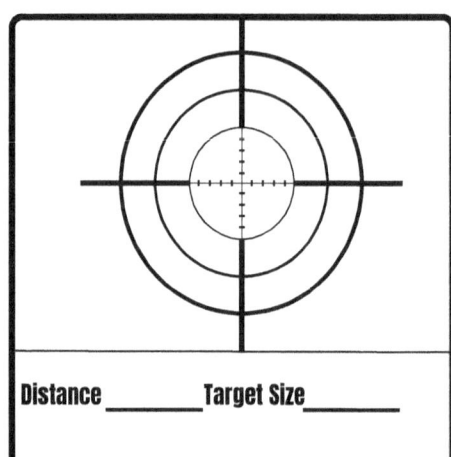
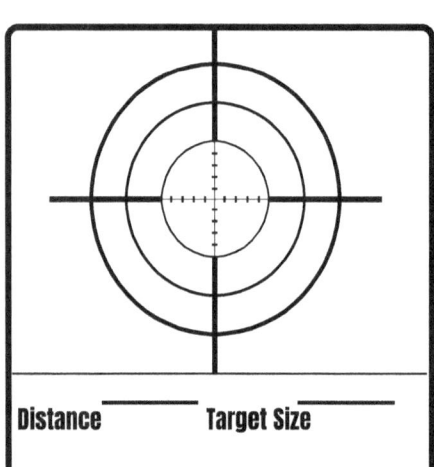
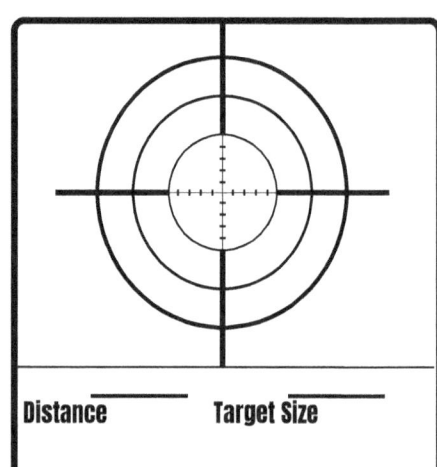
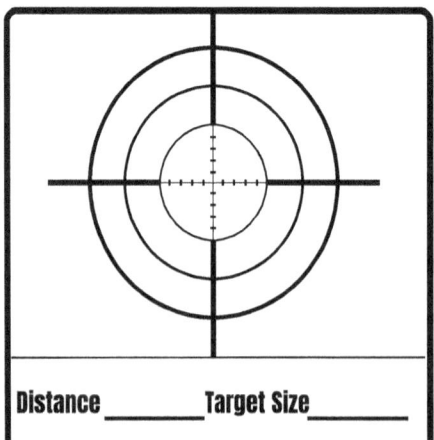
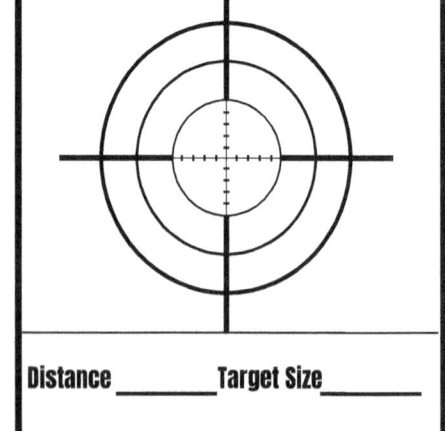

📅 Date	
⏱ Time	
📍 Location	
👥 Partner	
🔫 Firearm	
🎯 Scope Type	
Bullet Type	
Powder	
Primer	
Brass	
Seating Depth	

Light Conditions

Bright 1 2 3 4 5 Dark

Rating

Weapon Hanling	☆☆☆☆☆
Hit Rate	☆☆☆☆☆
Overall Results	☆☆☆☆☆

Session Highlights

Additional Notes

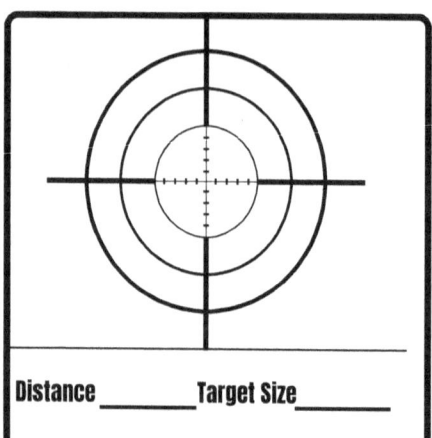

Distance _____ Target Size _____

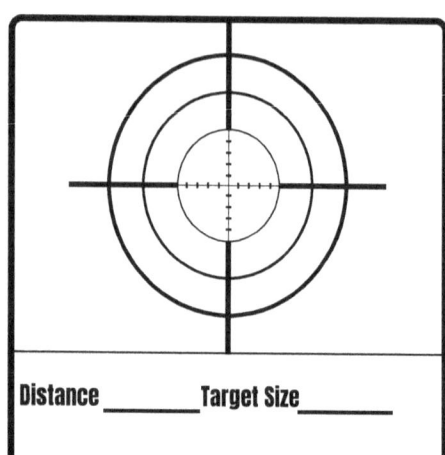

Distance _____ Target Size _____

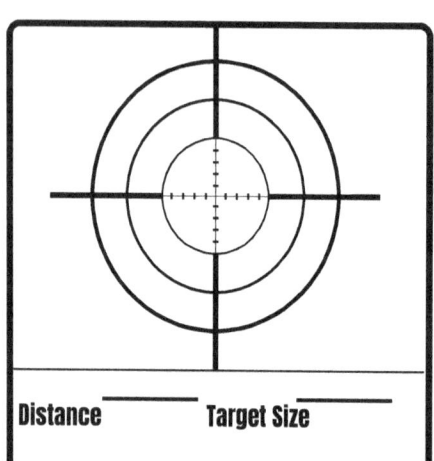

Distance _____ Target Size _____

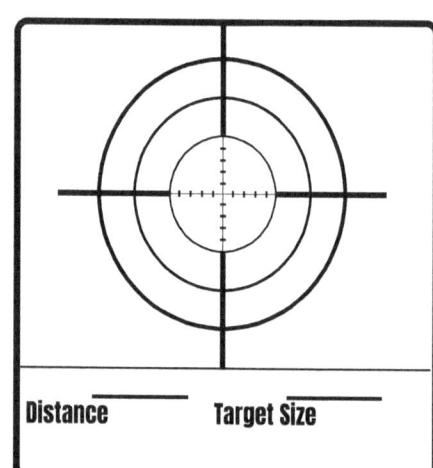

Distance _____ Target Size _____

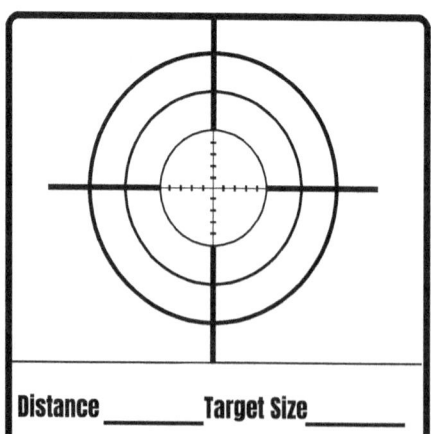

Distance _____ Target Size _____

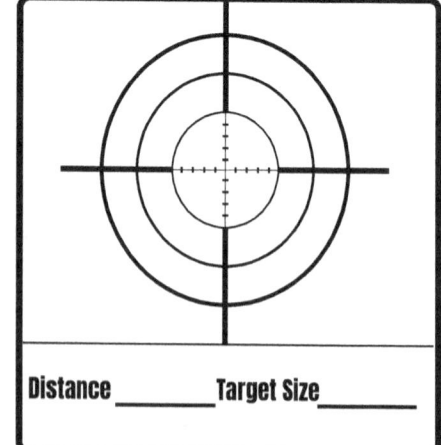

Distance _____ Target Size _____

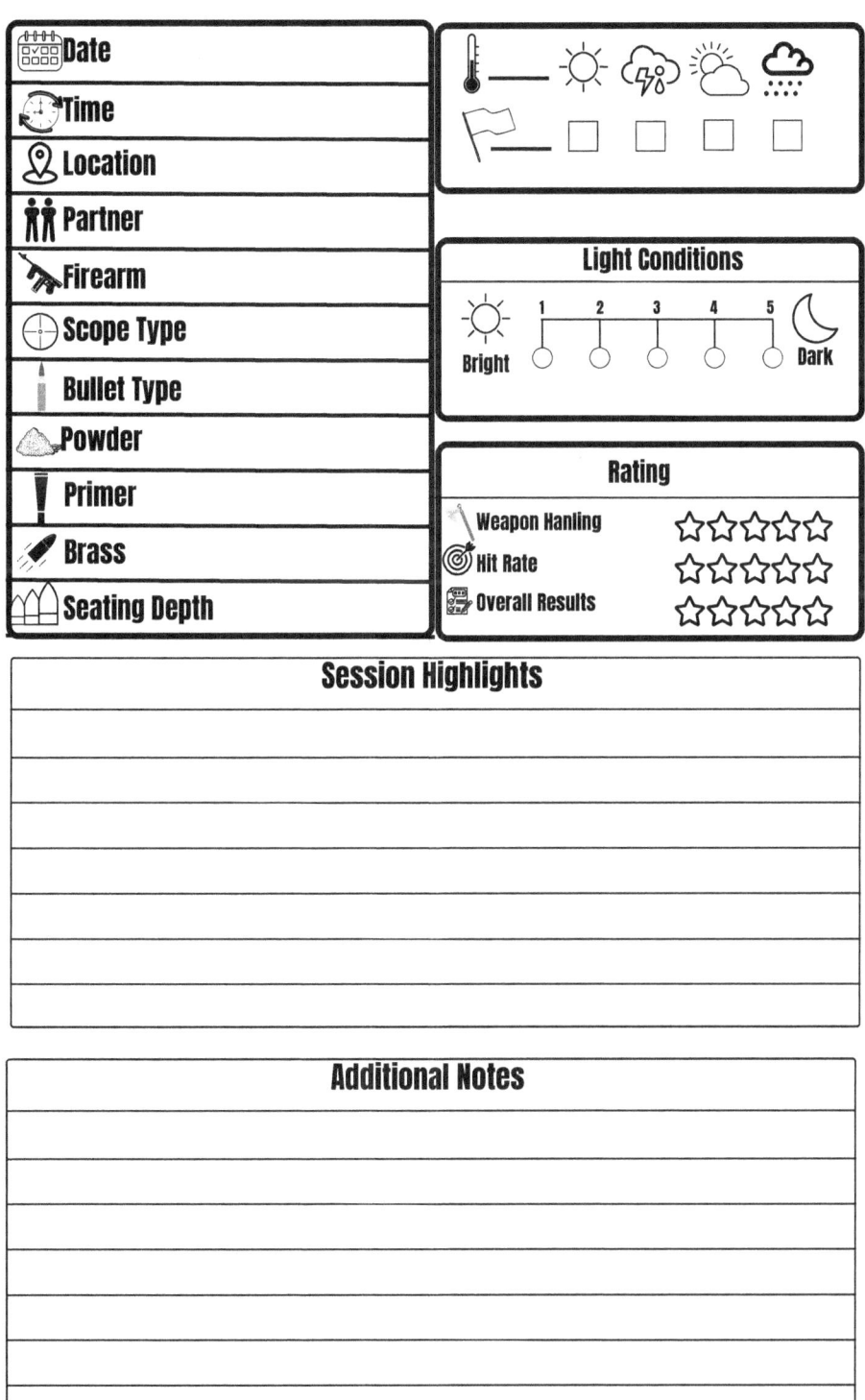

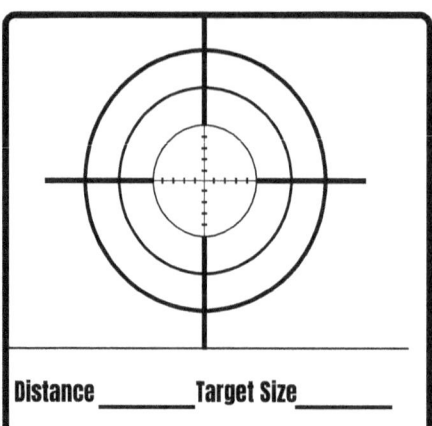
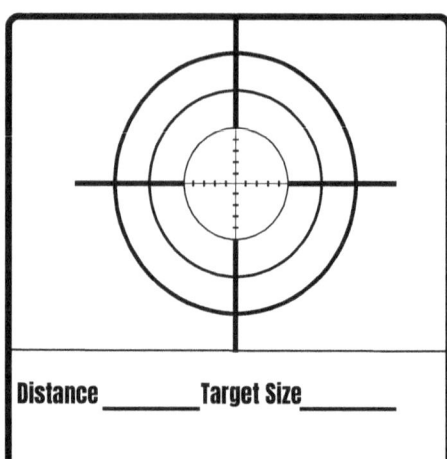
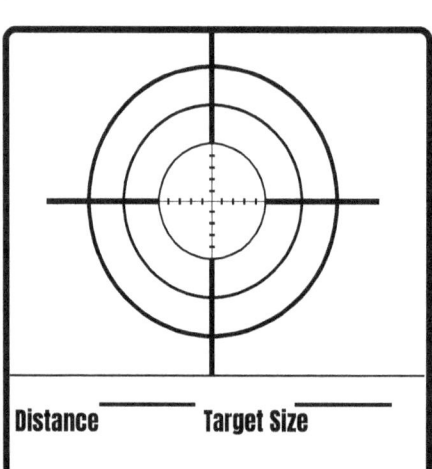
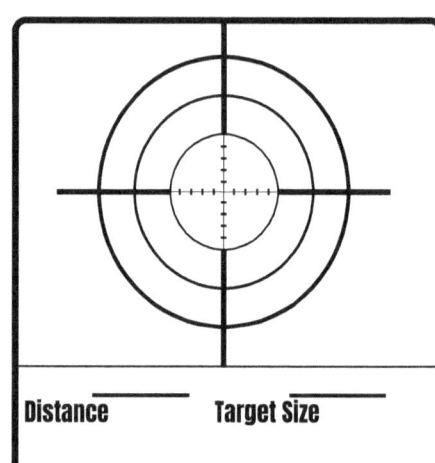
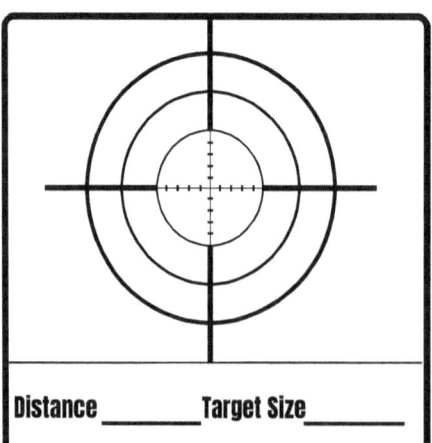
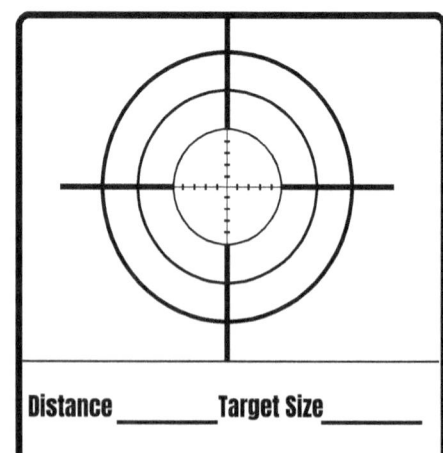

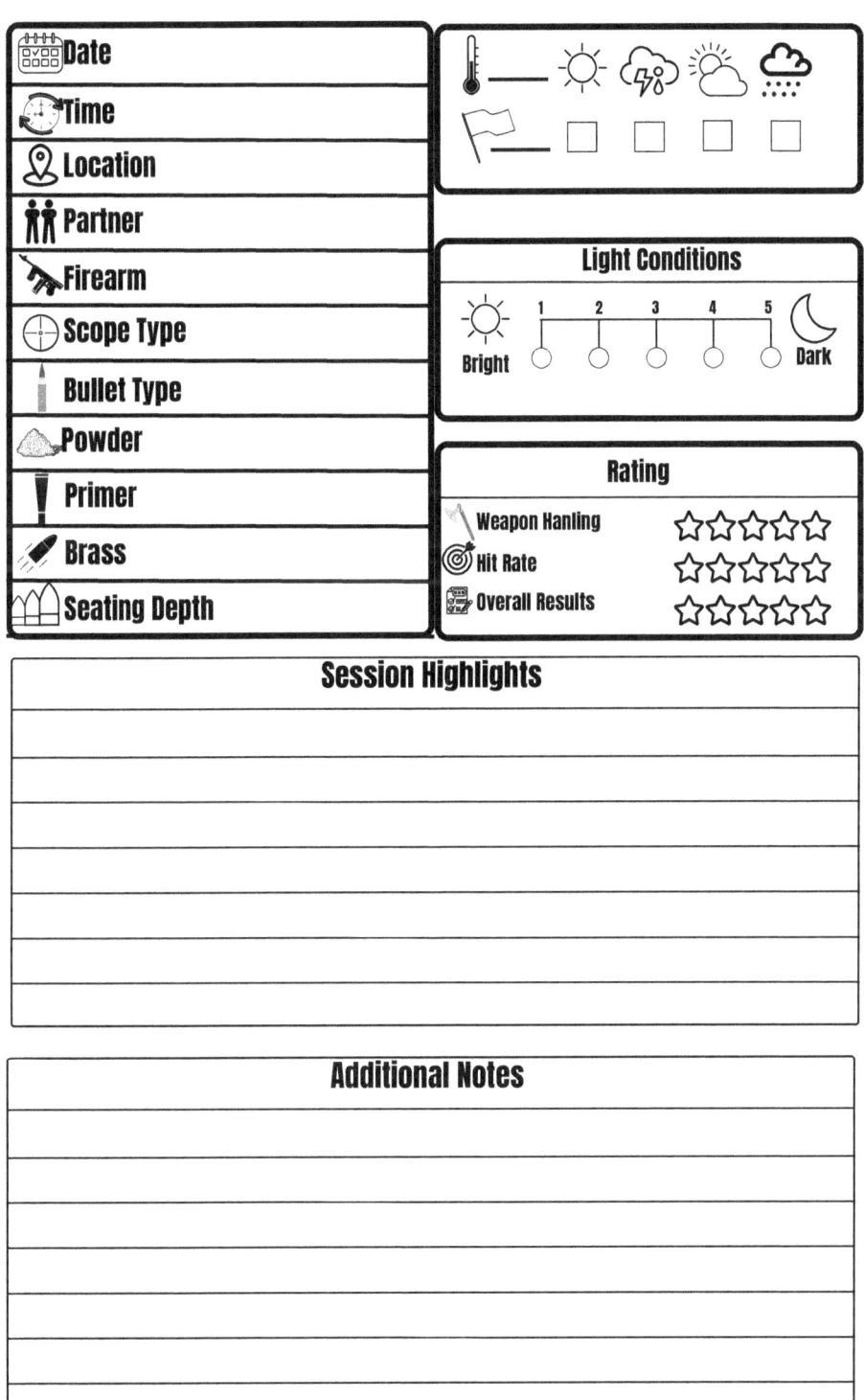

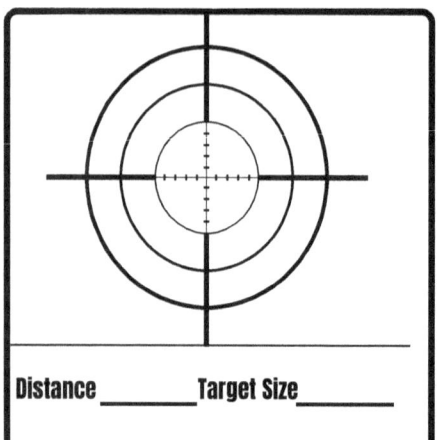
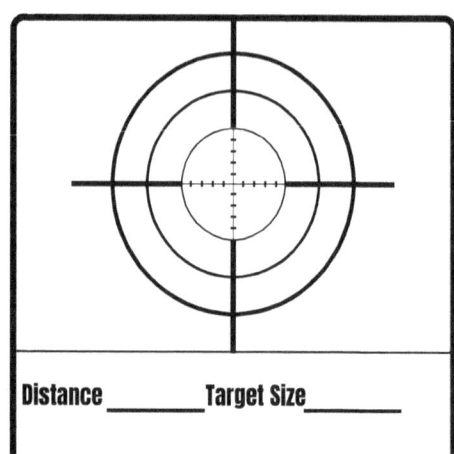
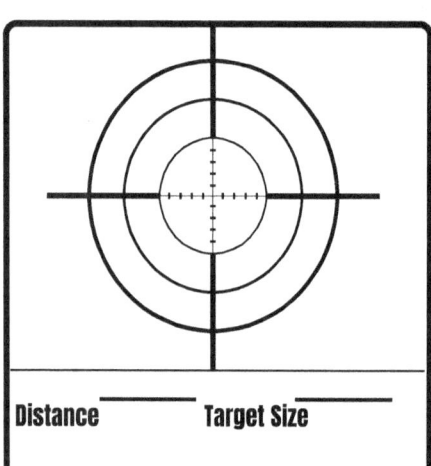
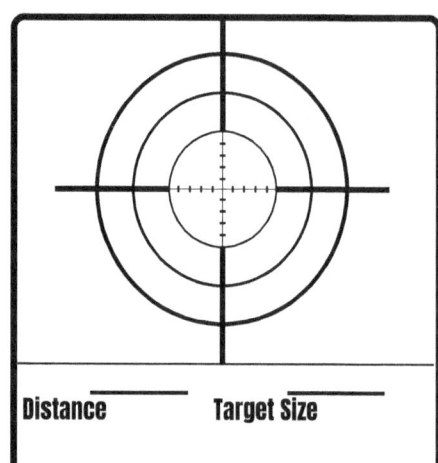
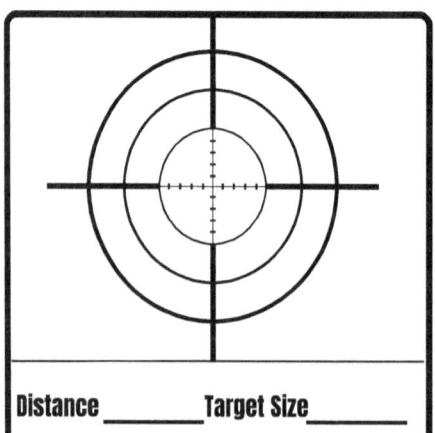
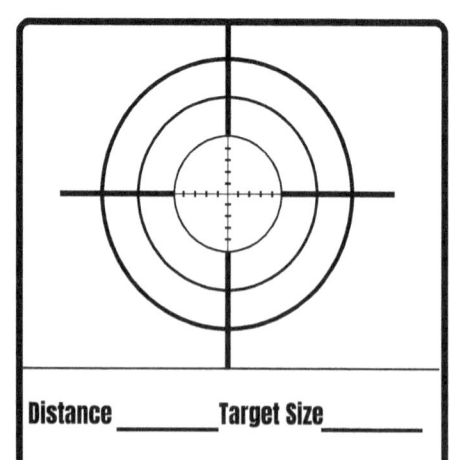

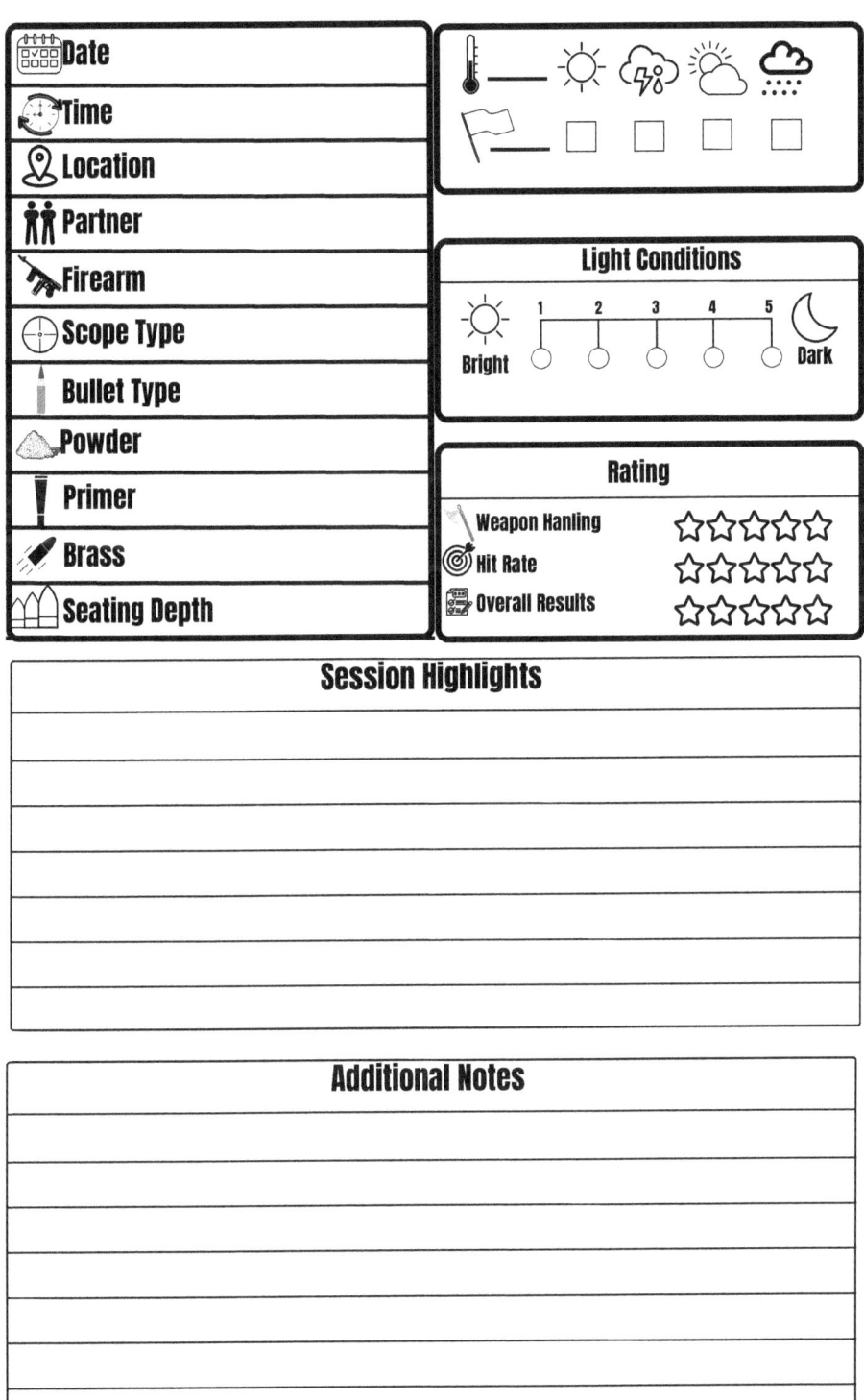

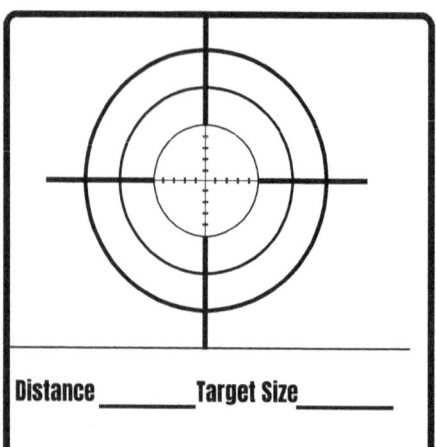

Distance _____ Target Size _____

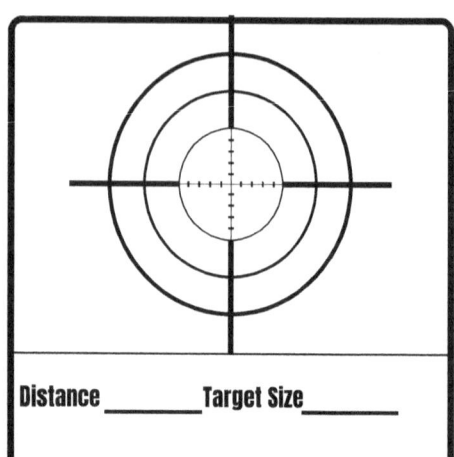

Distance _____ Target Size _____

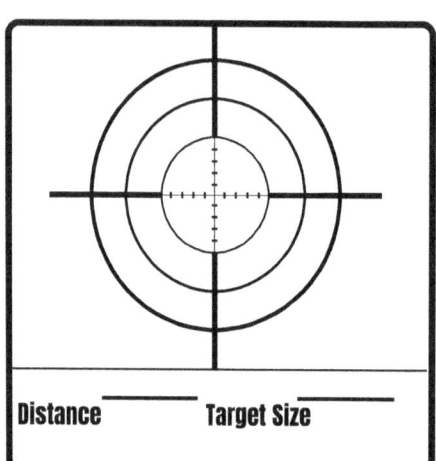

Distance _____ Target Size _____

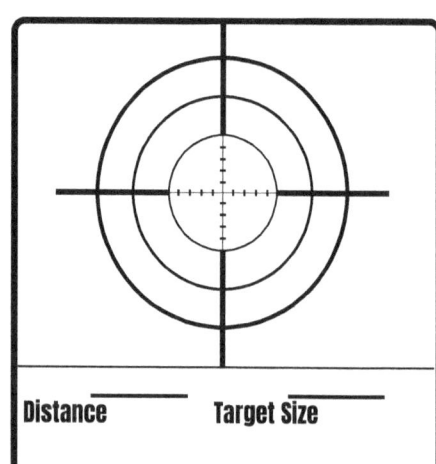

Distance _____ Target Size _____

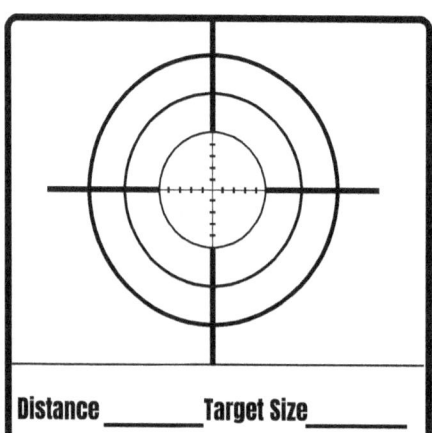

Distance _____ Target Size _____

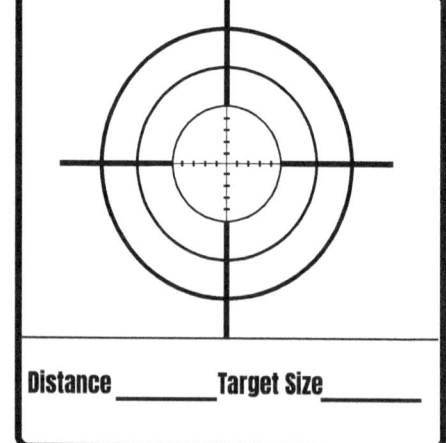

Distance _____ Target Size _____

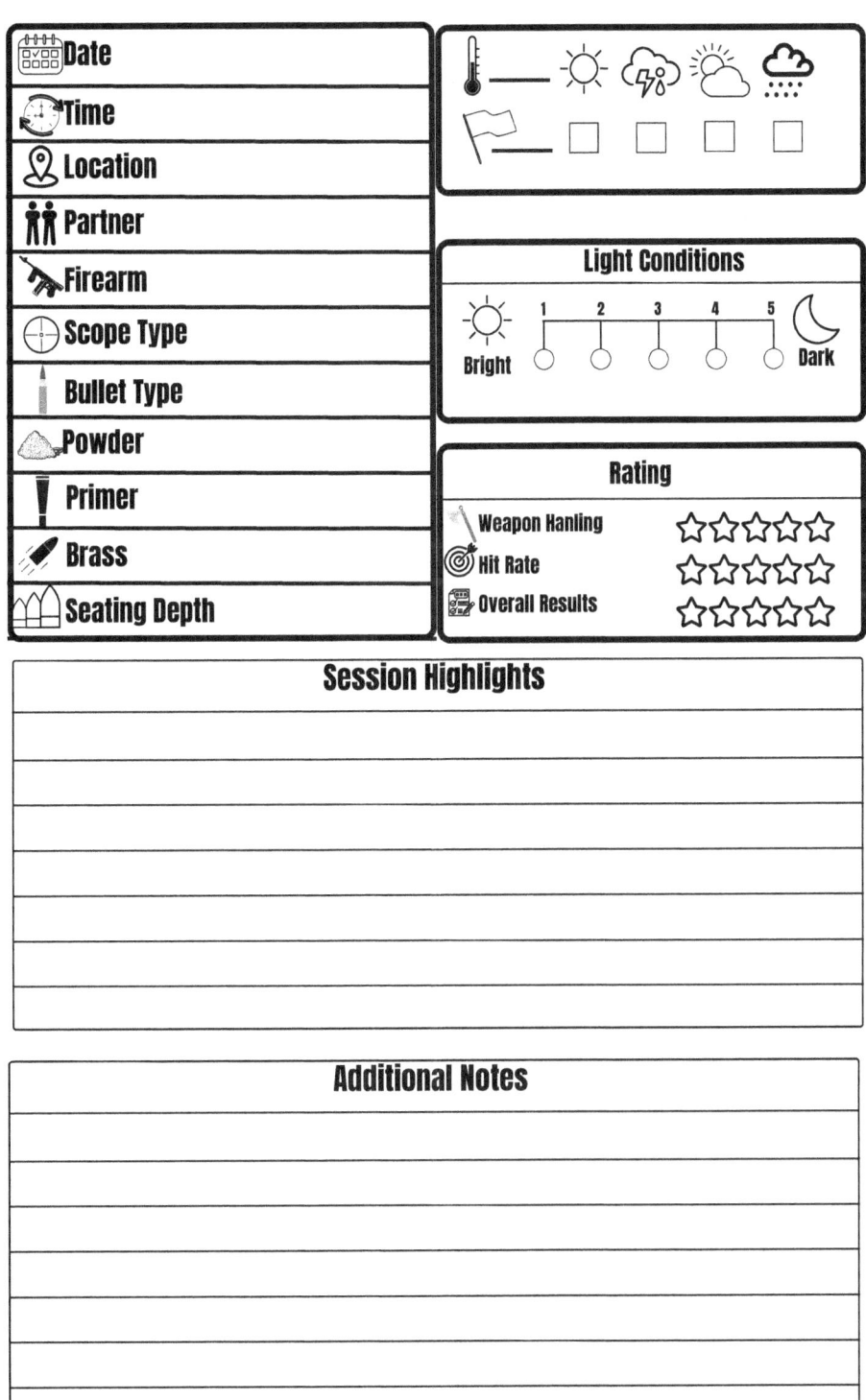

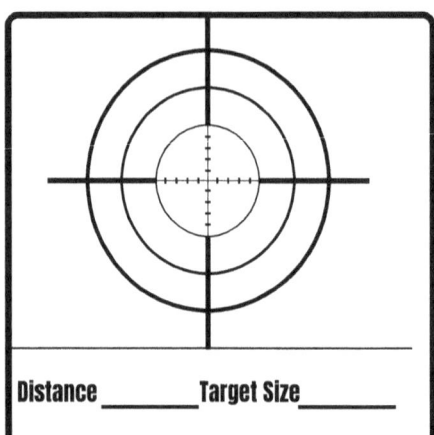
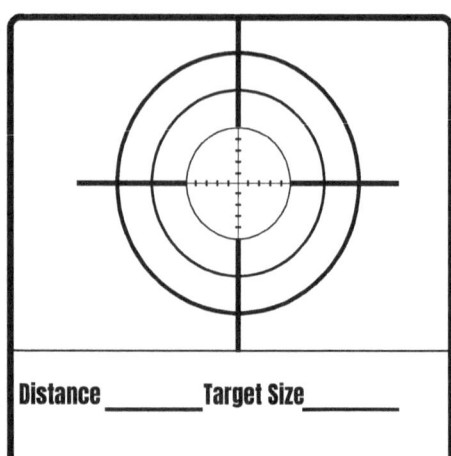
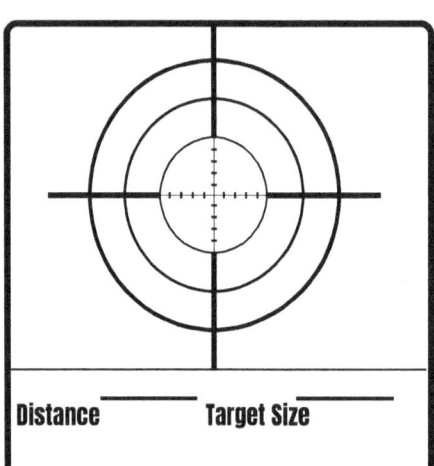
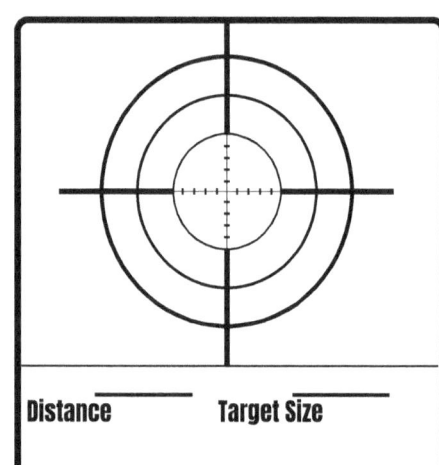
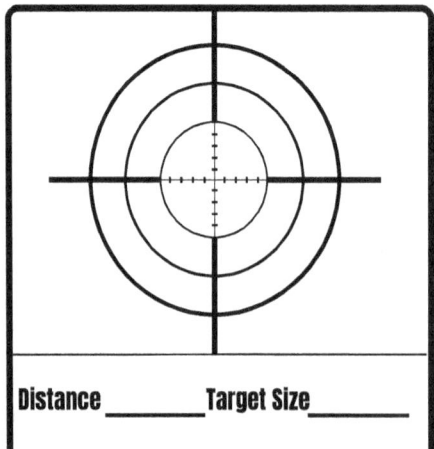
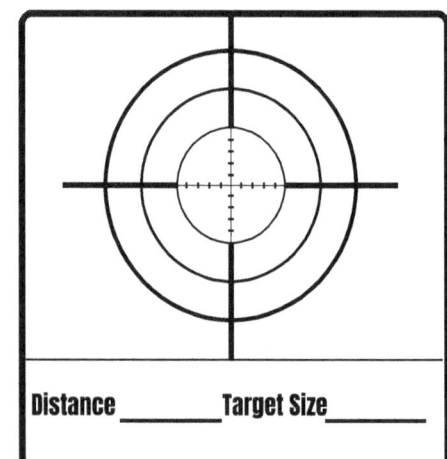

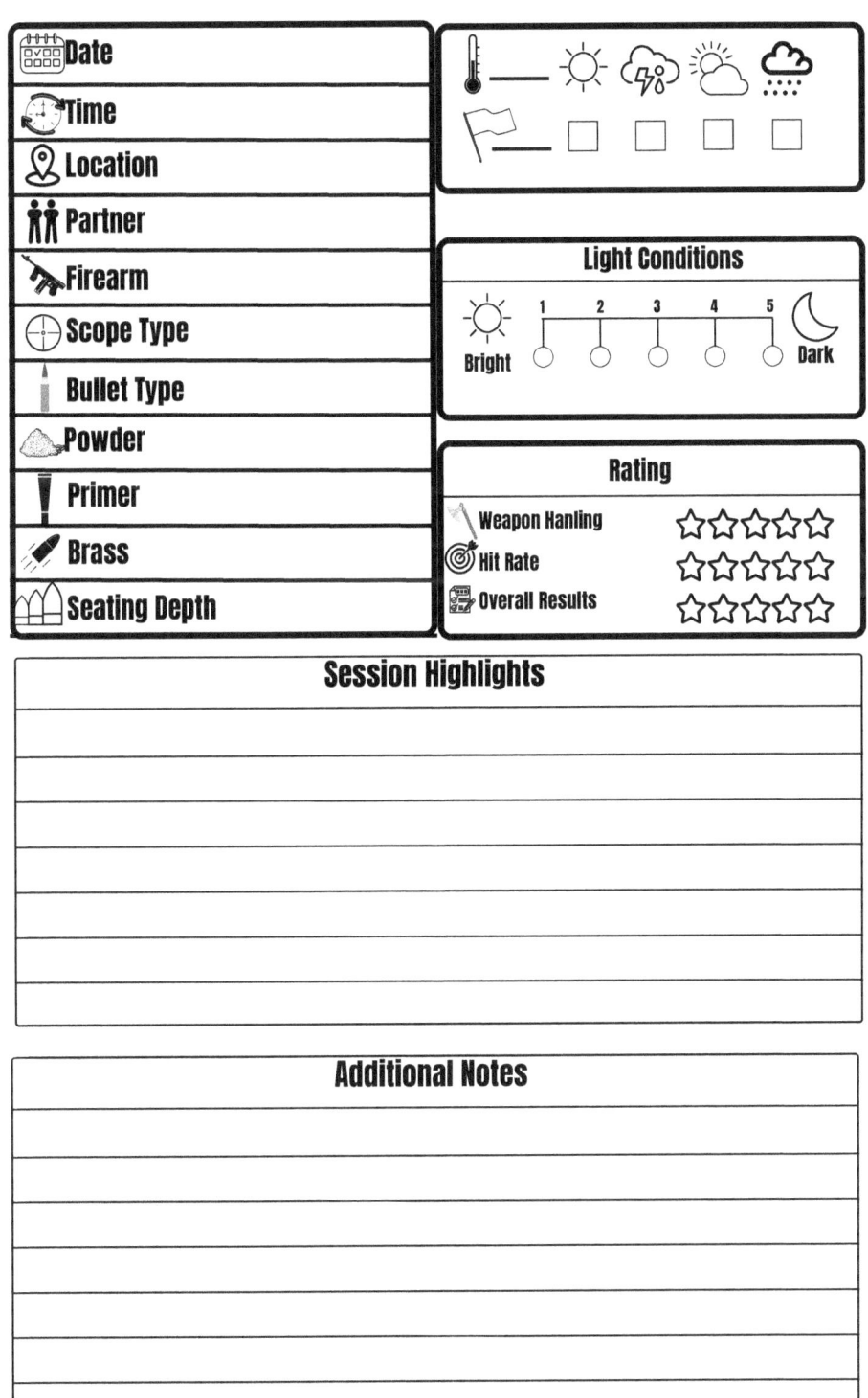

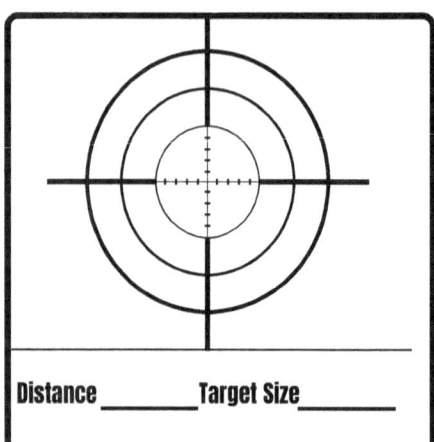

Distance _____ Target Size _____

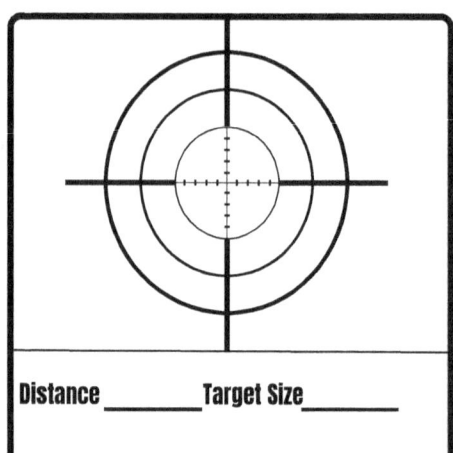

Distance _____ Target Size _____

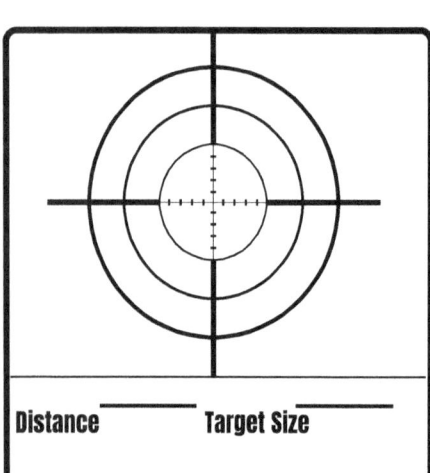

Distance _____ Target Size _____

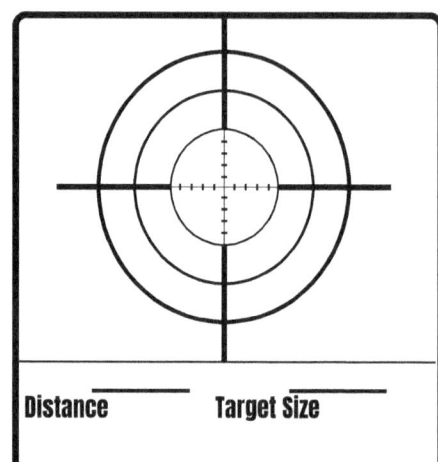

Distance _____ Target Size _____

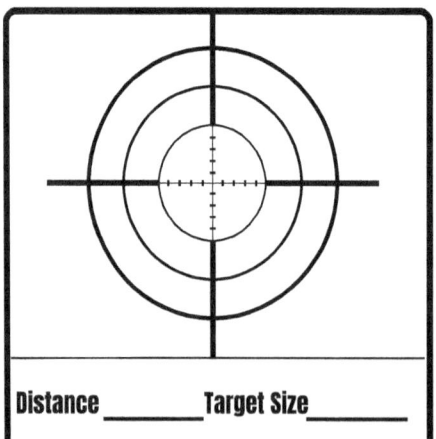

Distance _____ Target Size _____

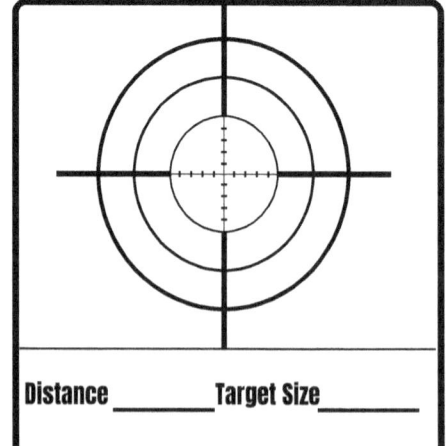

Distance _____ Target Size _____

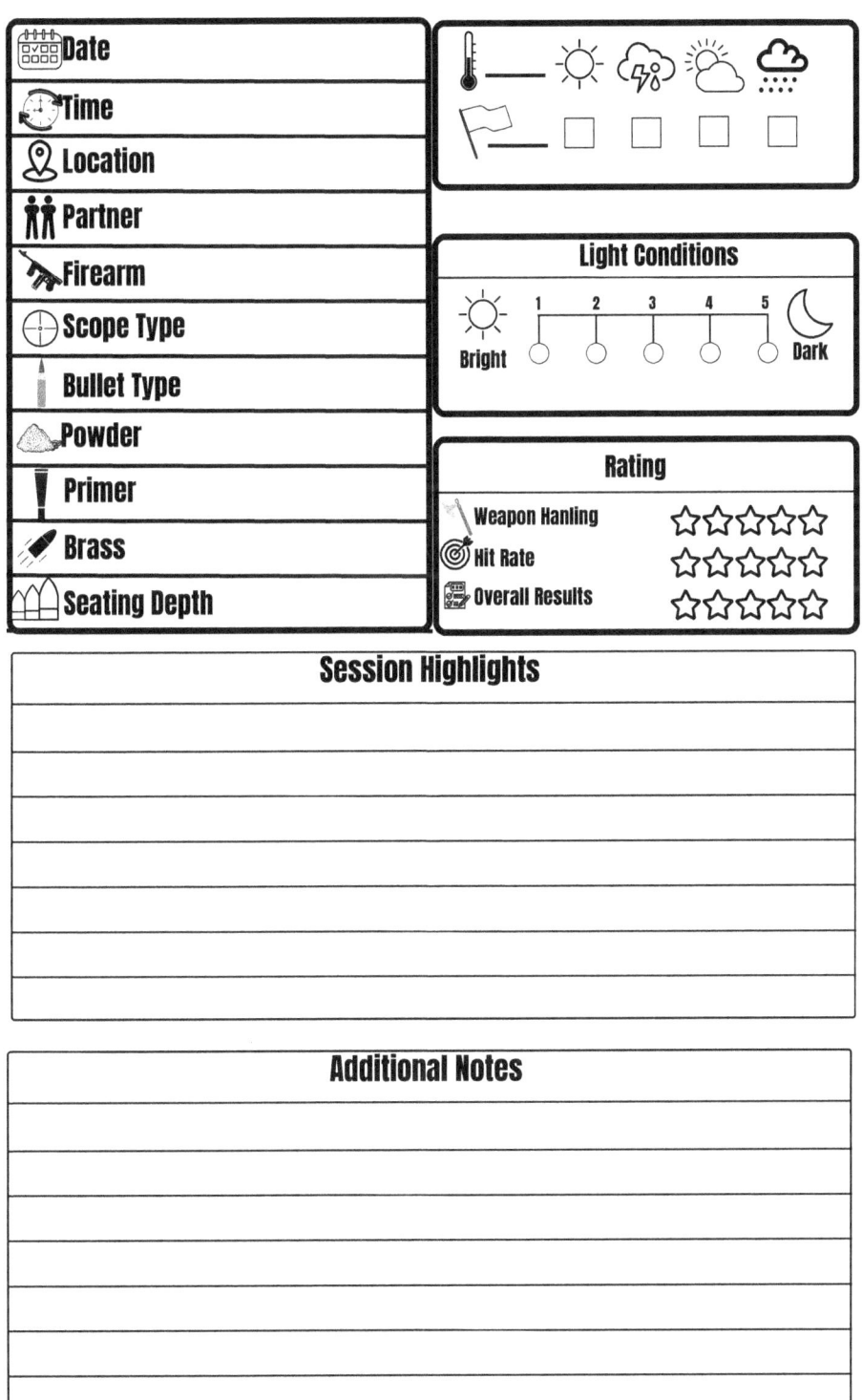

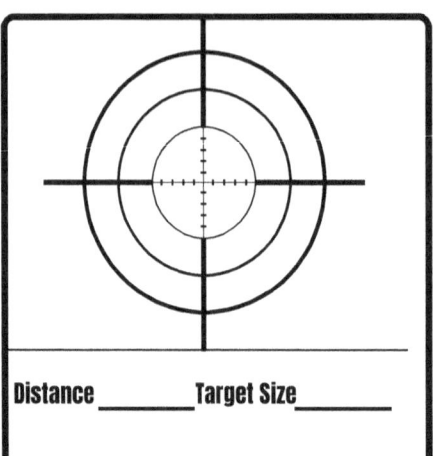
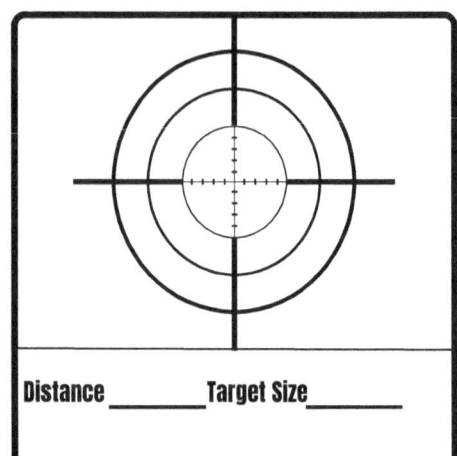
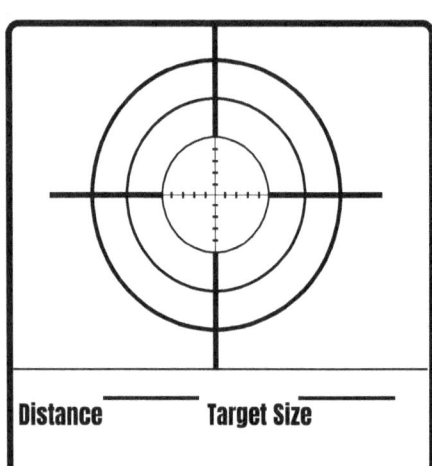
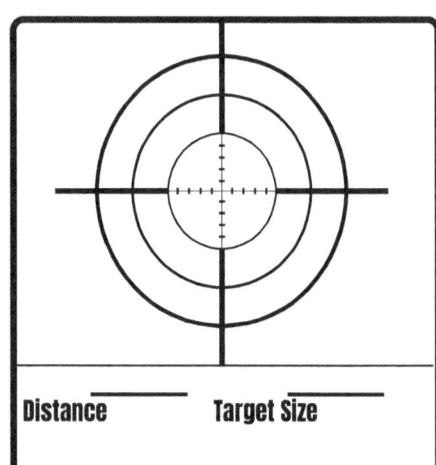
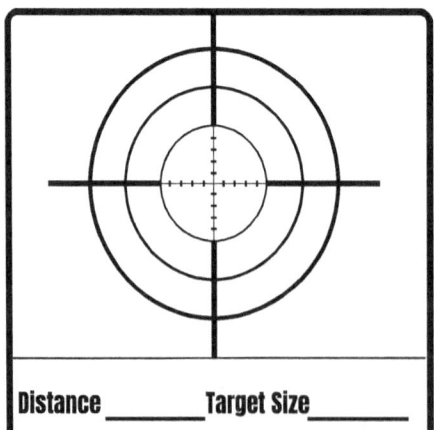
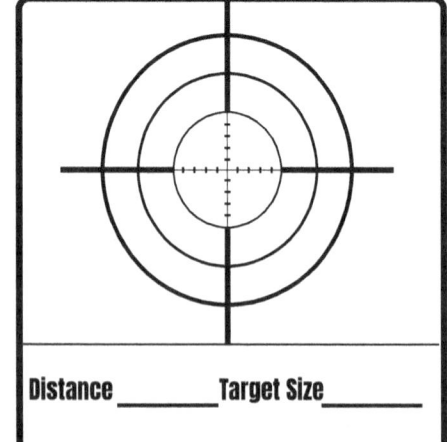

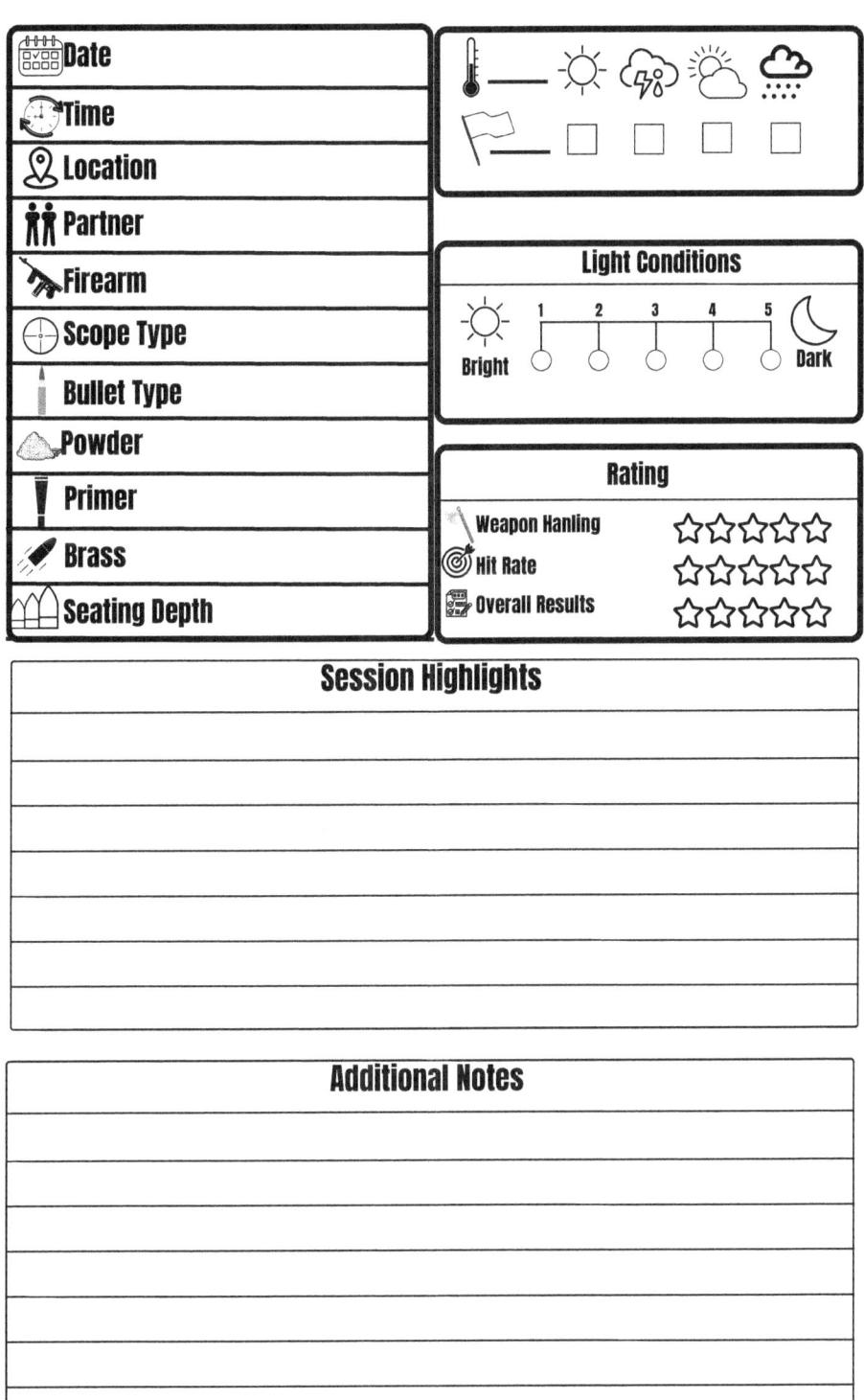

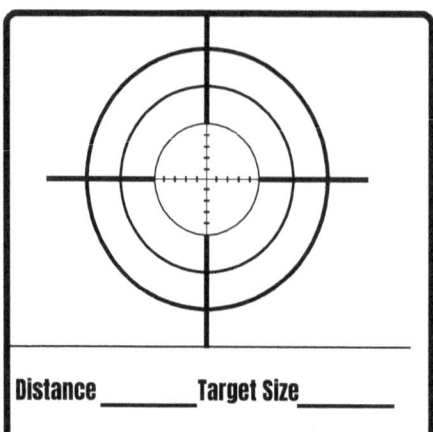
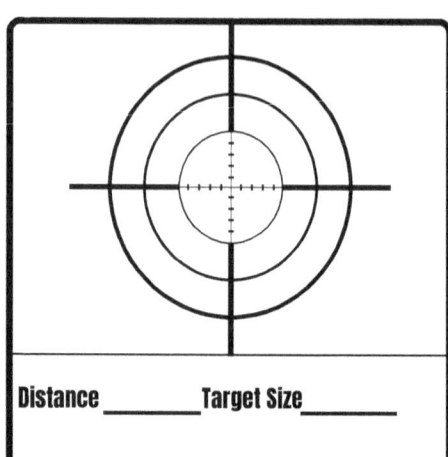
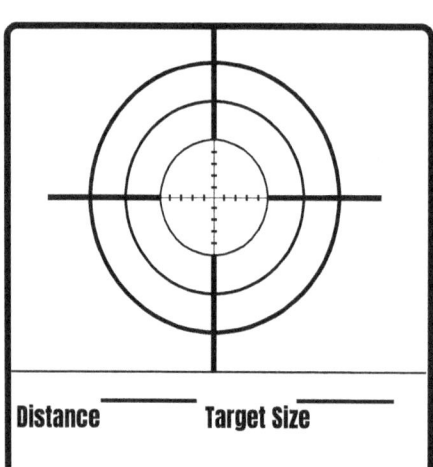
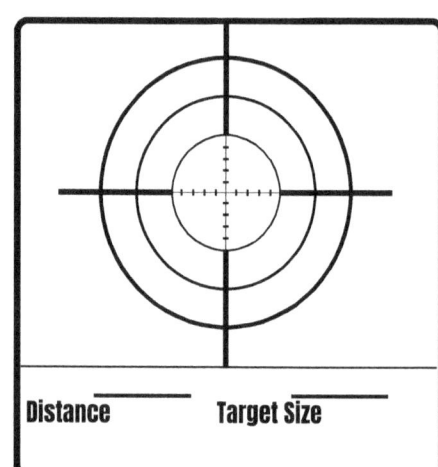
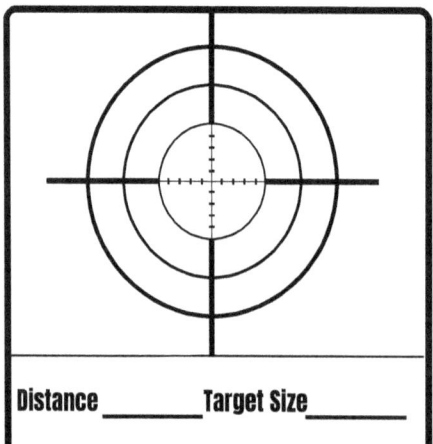
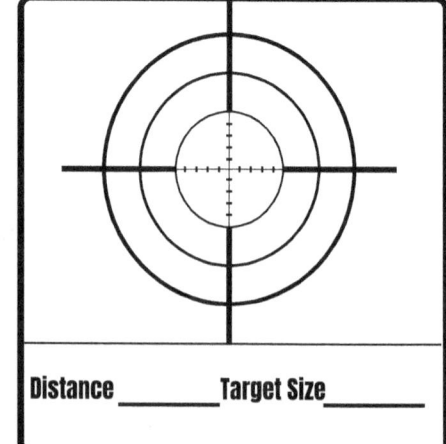

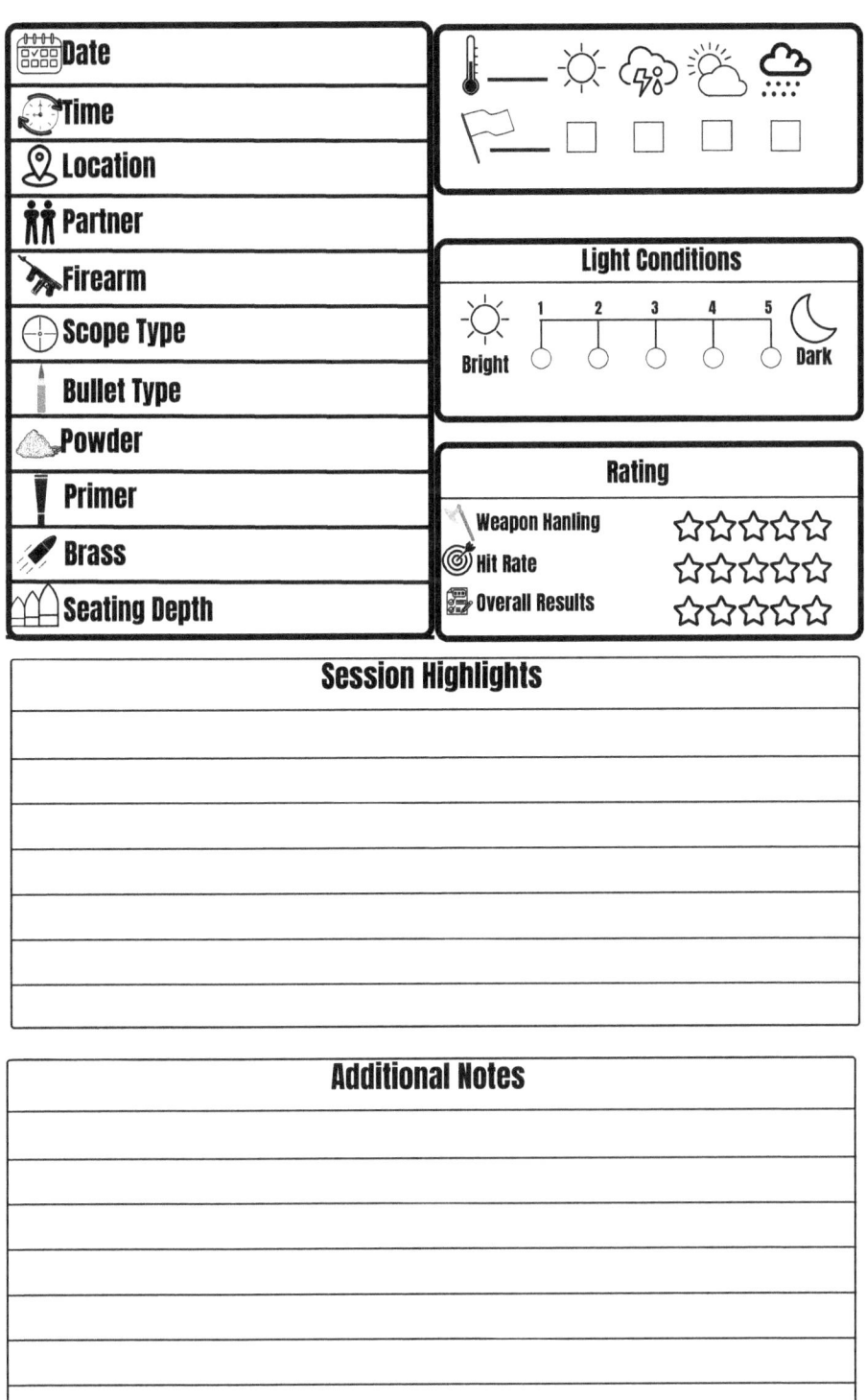

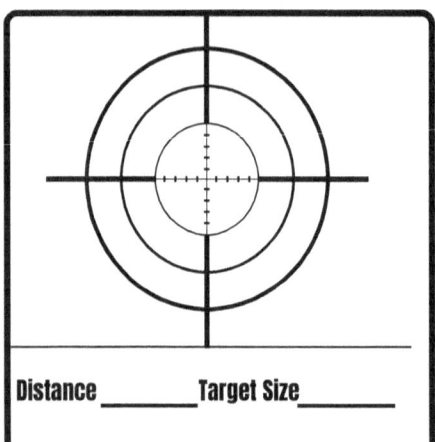

Distance _____ Target Size _____

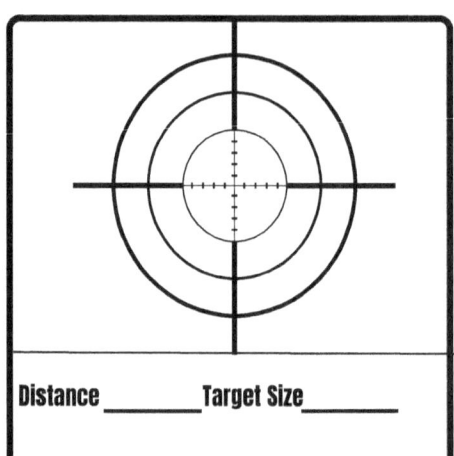

Distance _____ Target Size _____

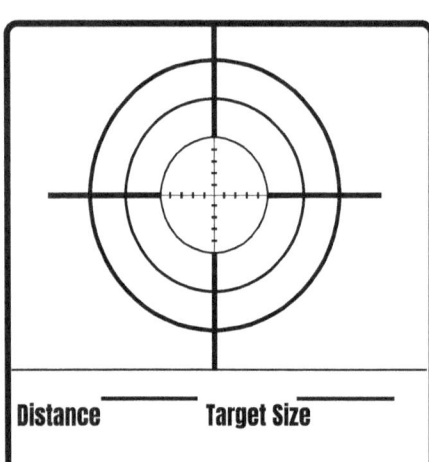

Distance _____ Target Size _____

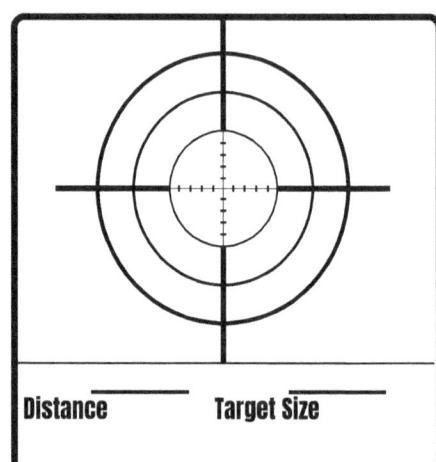

Distance _____ Target Size _____

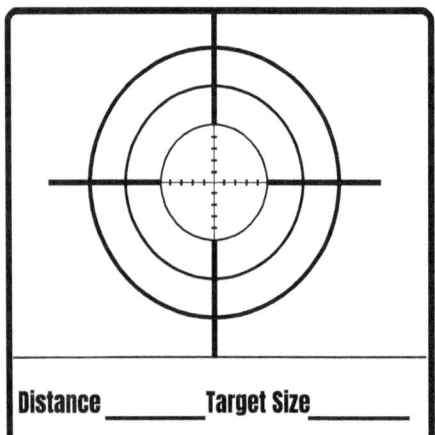

Distance _____ Target Size _____

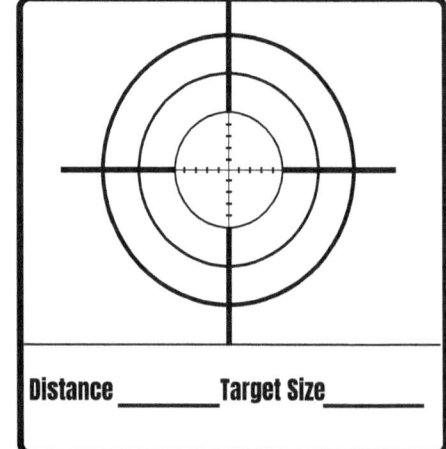

Distance _____ Target Size _____

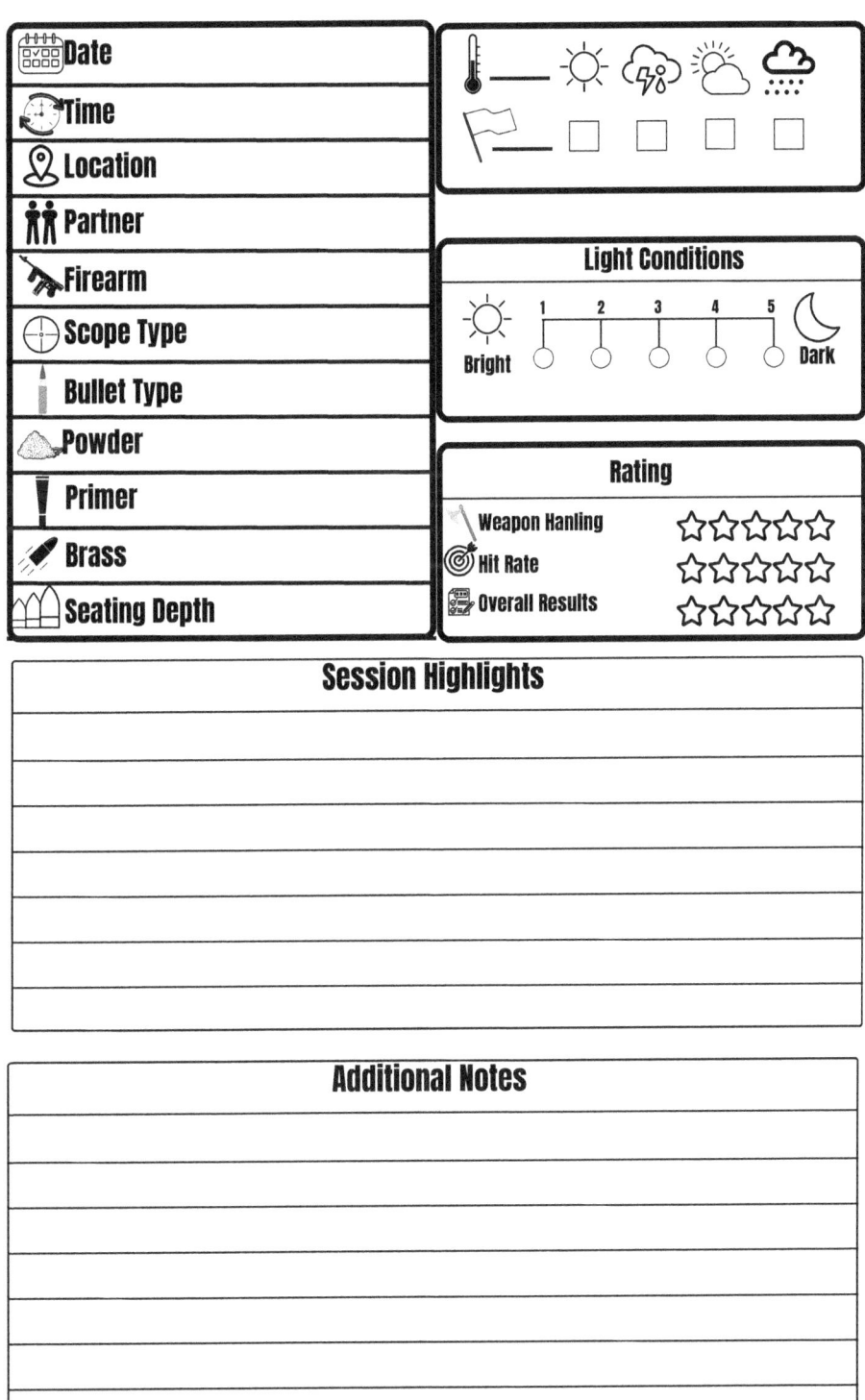

Date	
Time	
Location	
Partner	
Firearm	
Scope Type	
Bullet Type	
Powder	
Primer	
Brass	
Seating Depth	

Light Conditions

Bright 1 — 2 — 3 — 4 — 5 Dark

Rating

Weapon Hanling	☆☆☆☆☆
Hit Rate	☆☆☆☆☆
Overall Results	☆☆☆☆☆

Session Highlights

Additional Notes

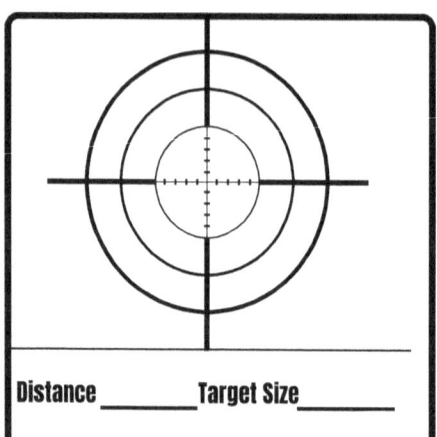
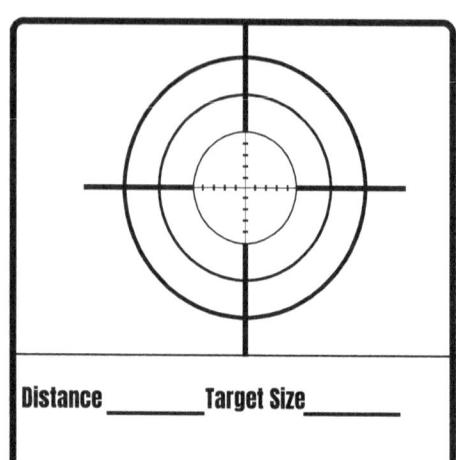
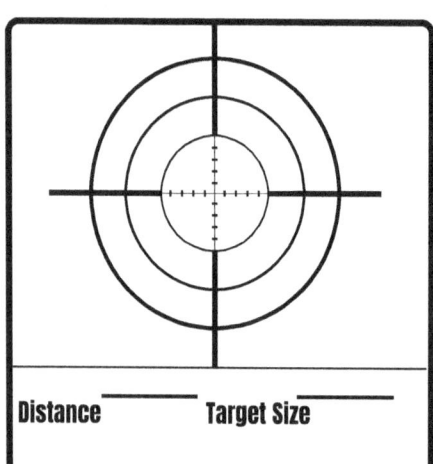
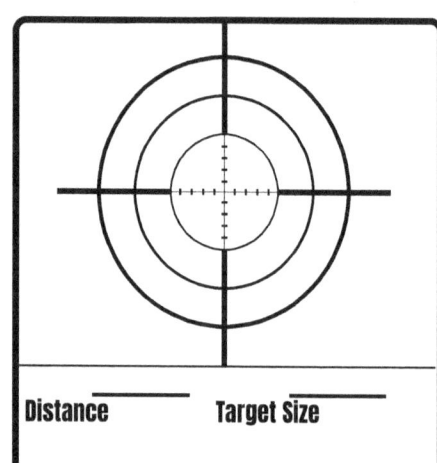
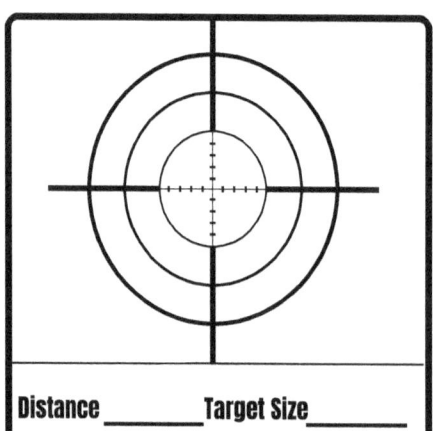
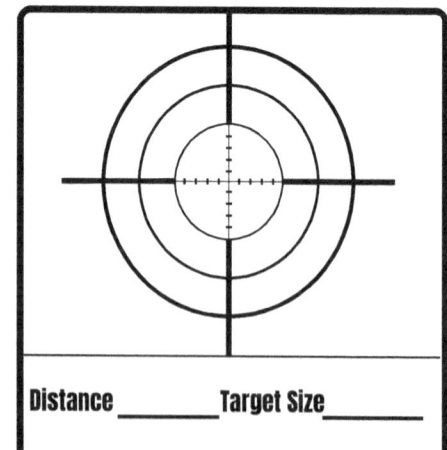

Date	
Time	
Location	
Partner	
Firearm	
Scope Type	
Bullet Type	
Powder	
Primer	
Brass	
Seating Depth	

Light Conditions

Bright 1 — 2 — 3 — 4 — 5 Dark

Rating

Weapon Hanling	☆☆☆☆☆
Hit Rate	☆☆☆☆☆
Overall Results	☆☆☆☆☆

Session Highlights

Additional Notes

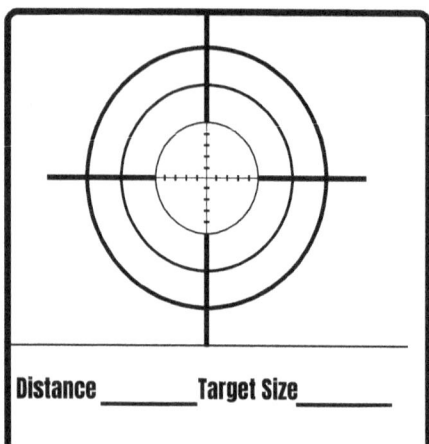
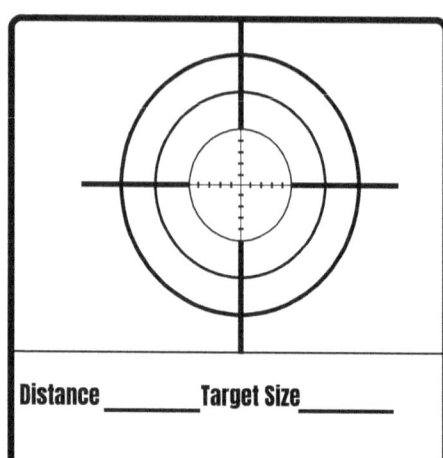
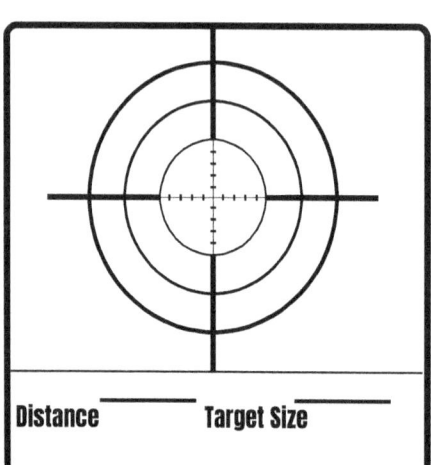
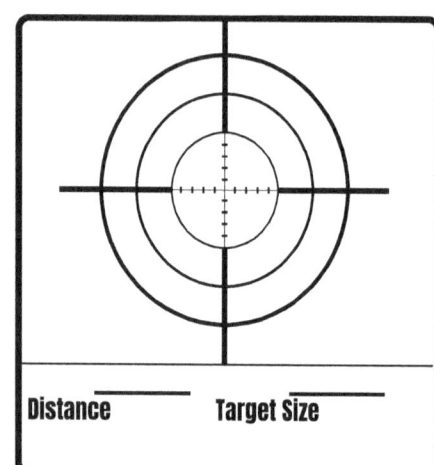
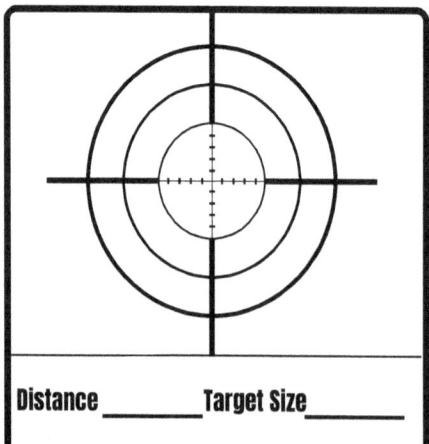
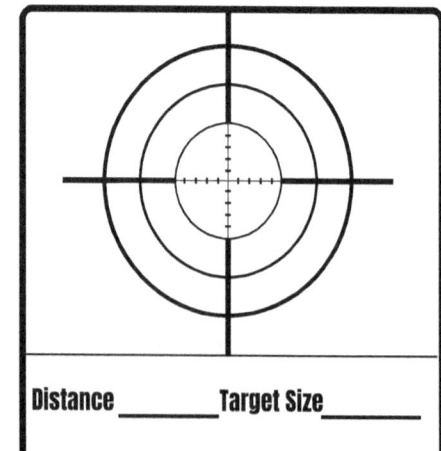

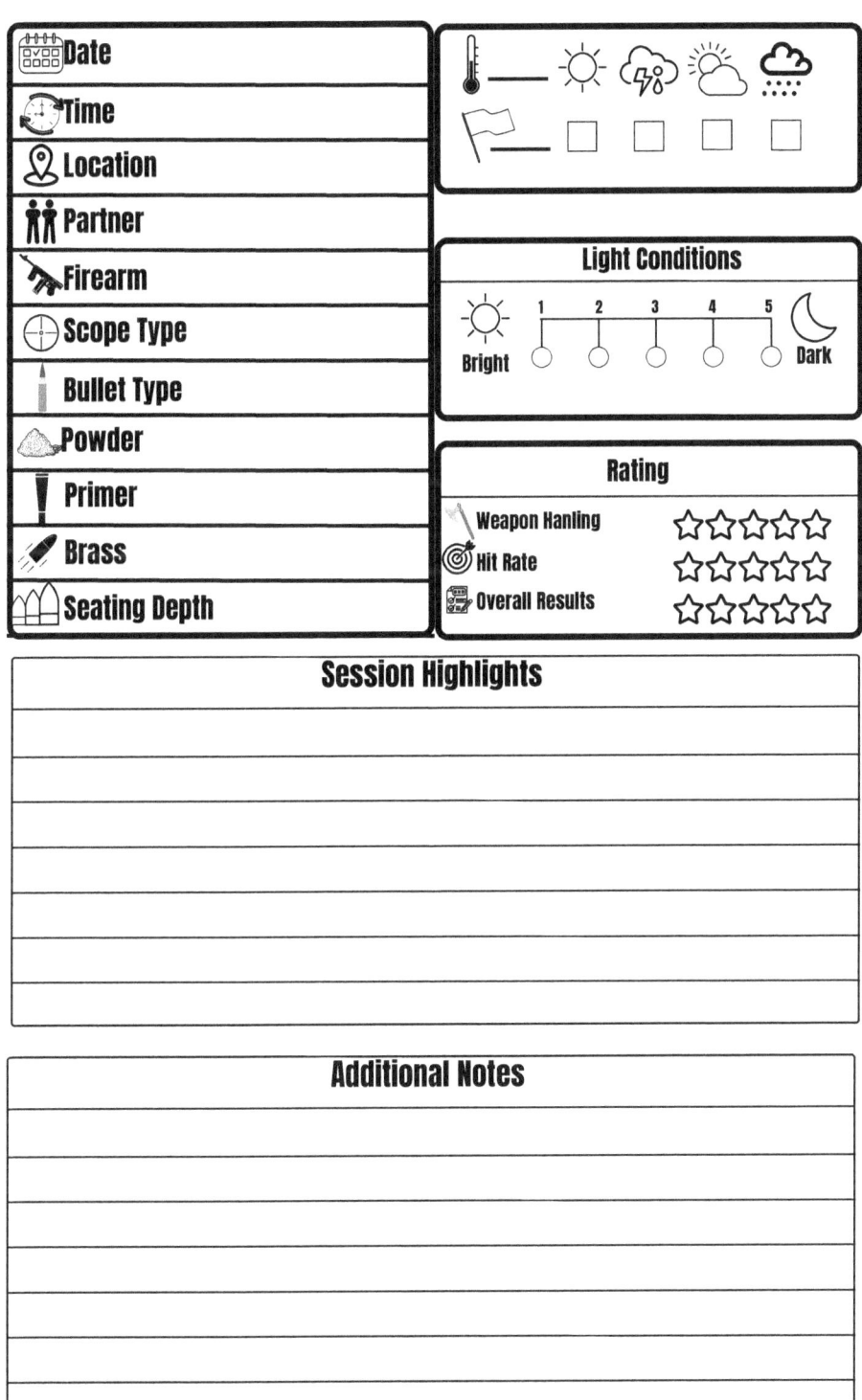

📅 Date	
⏱ Time	
📍 Location	
👥 Partner	
🔫 Firearm	
🔭 Scope Type	
Bullet Type	
Powder	
Primer	
Brass	
Seating Depth	

Light Conditions

Bright 1 — 2 — 3 — 4 — 5 Dark

Rating

- Weapon Hanling ☆☆☆☆☆
- Hit Rate ☆☆☆☆☆
- Overall Results ☆☆☆☆☆

Session Highlights

Additional Notes

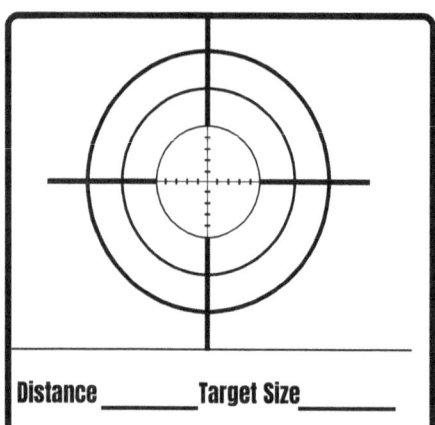
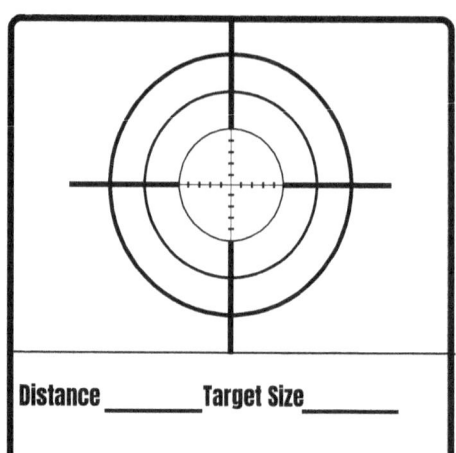
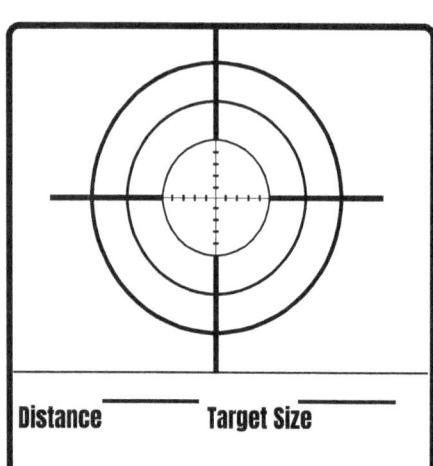
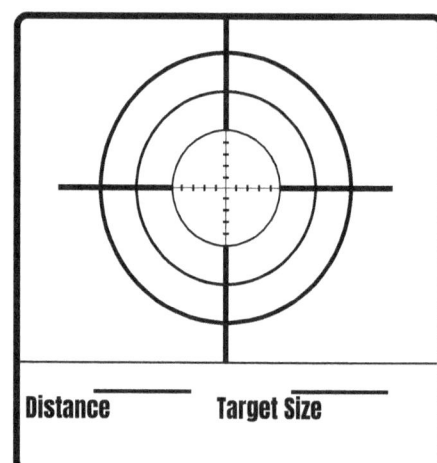
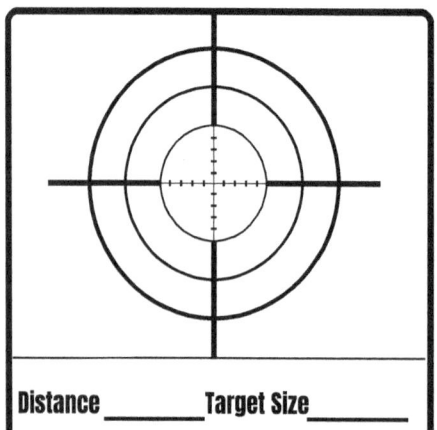
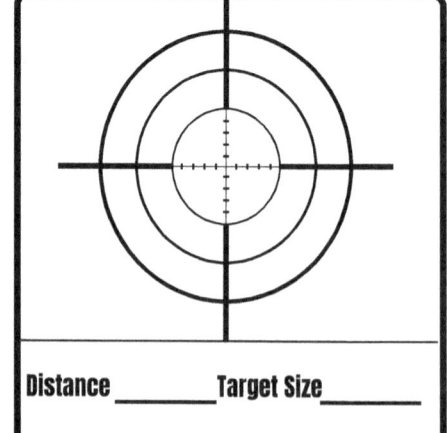

📅 Date	
⏱ Time	
📍 Location	
👥 Partner	
🔫 Firearm	
🔭 Scope Type	
Bullet Type	
Powder	
Primer	
Brass	
Seating Depth	

Light Conditions
Bright ☀ 1 — 2 — 3 — 4 — 5 ☾ Dark

Rating
- Weapon Hanling ☆☆☆☆☆
- Hit Rate ☆☆☆☆☆
- Overall Results ☆☆☆☆☆

Session Highlights

―
―
―
―
―
―
―
―
―

Additional Notes

―
―
―
―
―
―
―
―
―

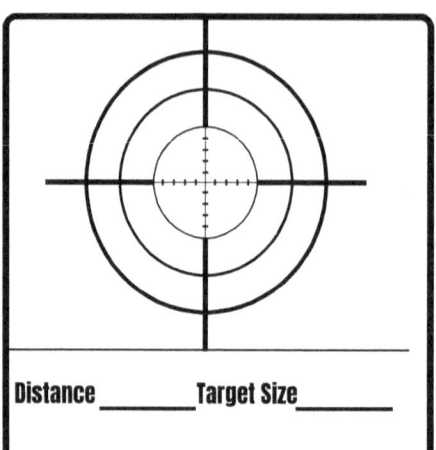
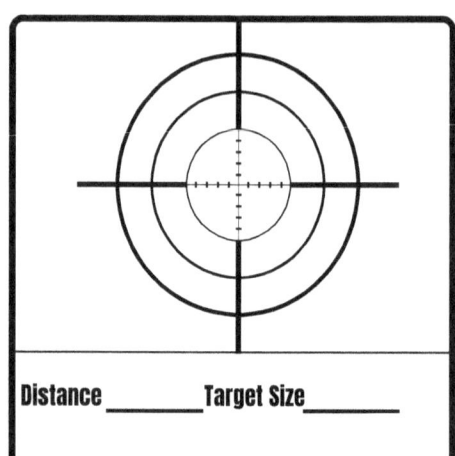
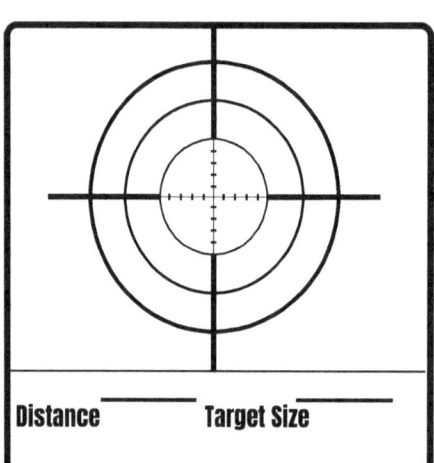
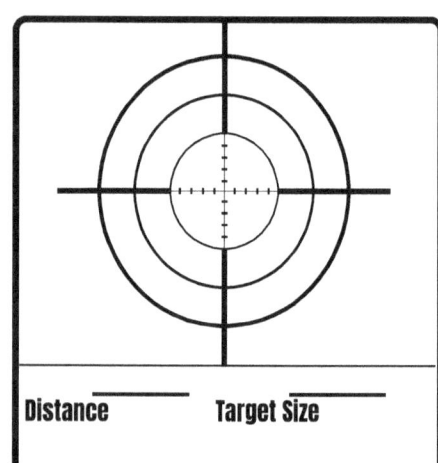
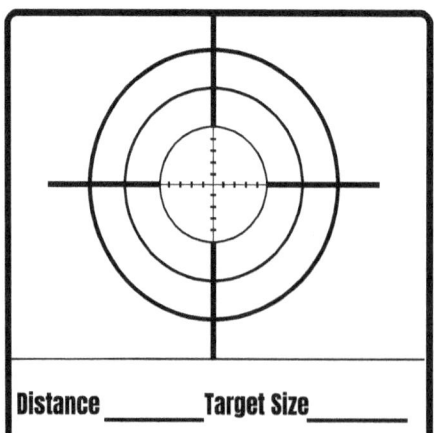
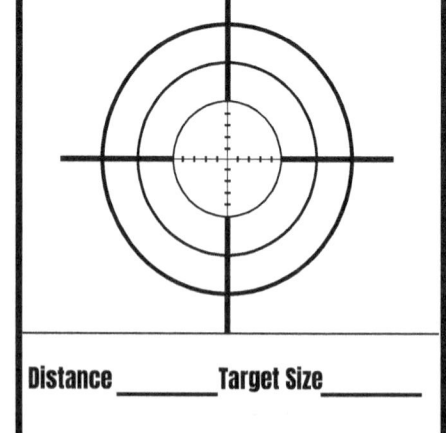

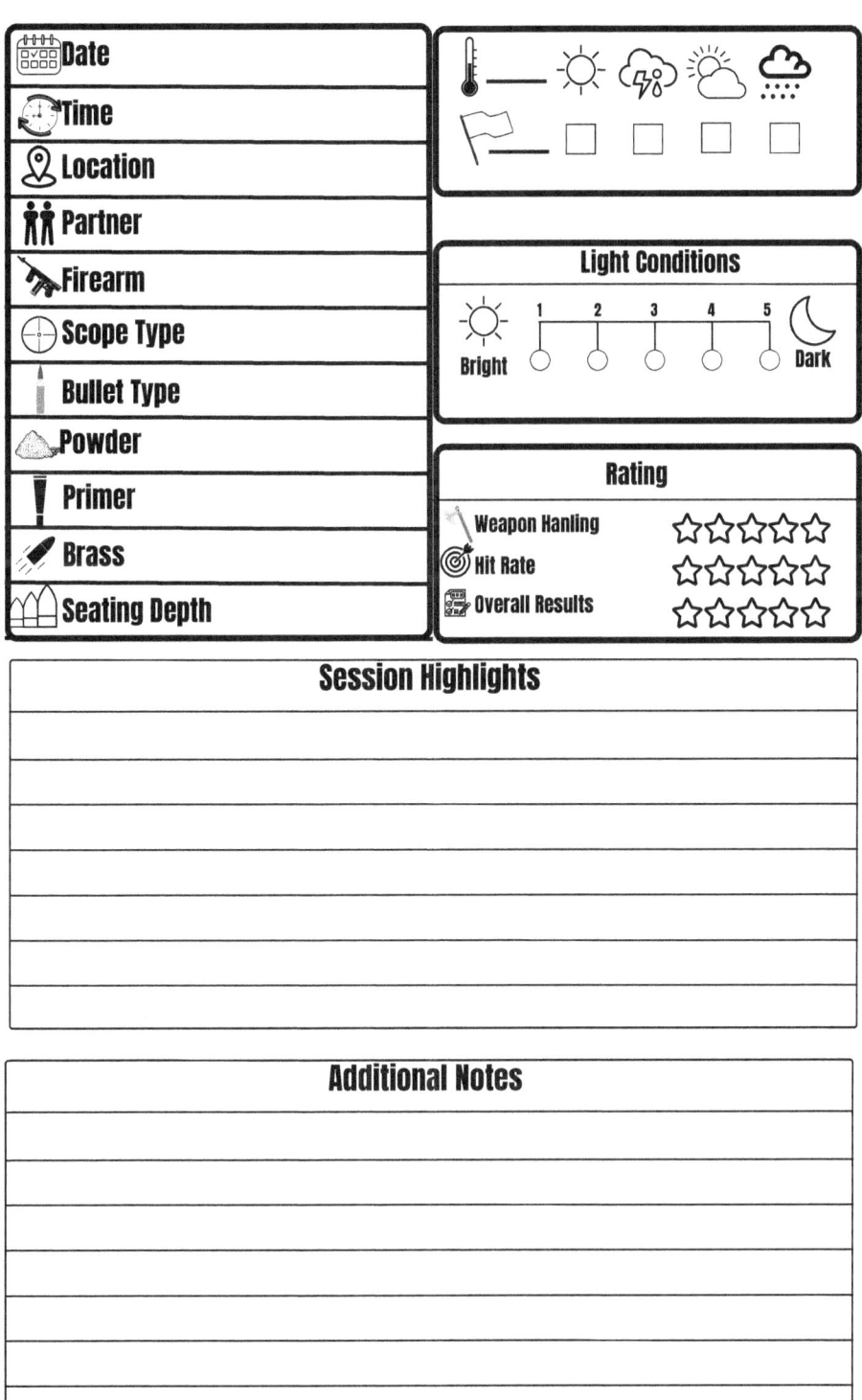

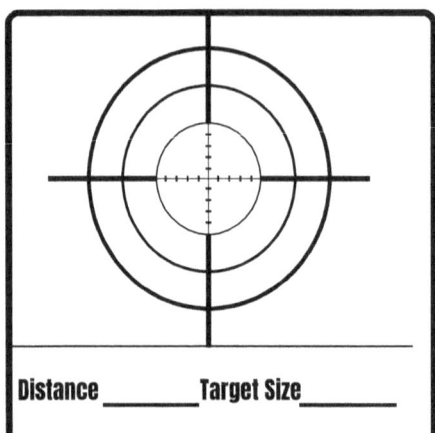
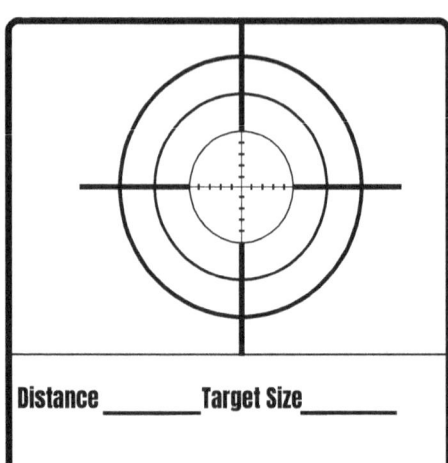
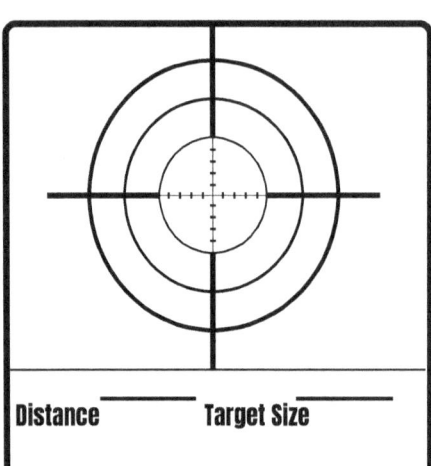
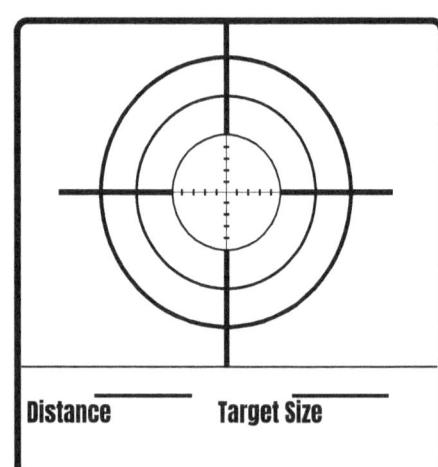
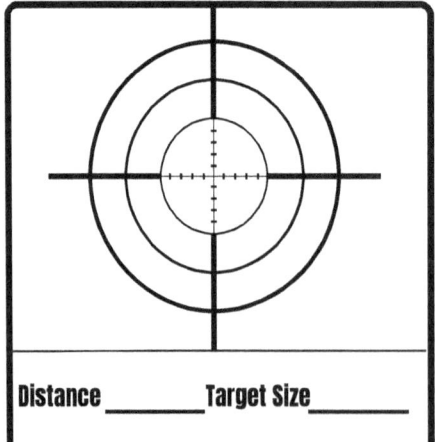
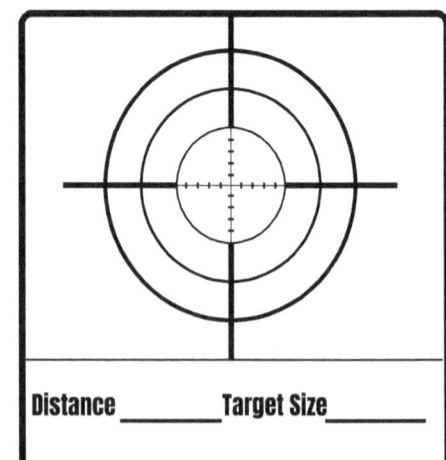

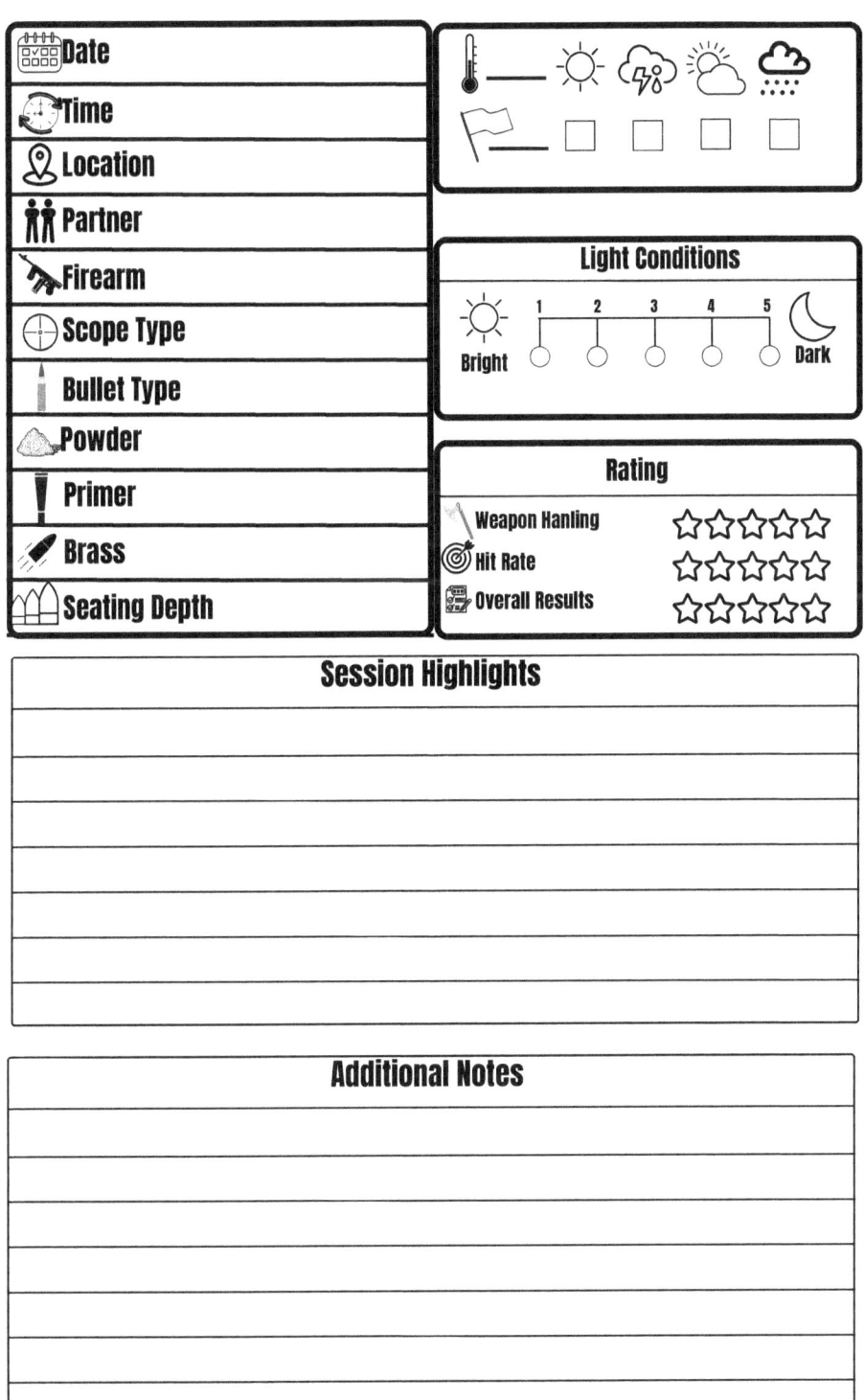

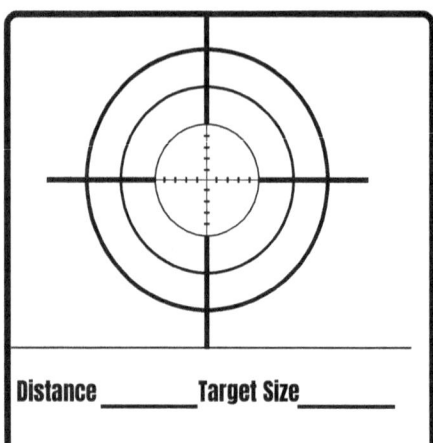

Distance _____ Target Size _____

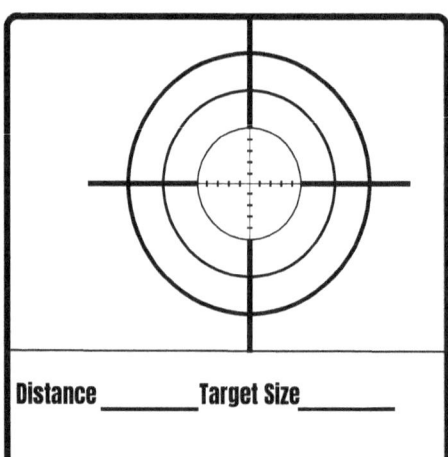

Distance _____ Target Size _____

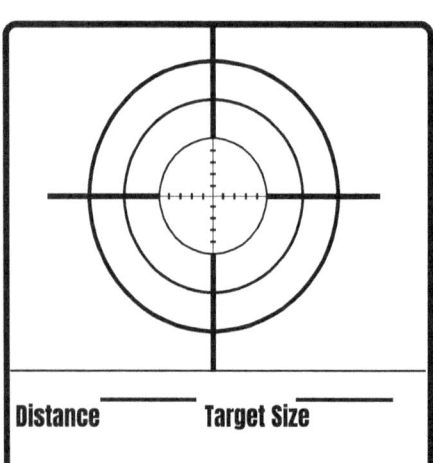

Distance _____ Target Size _____

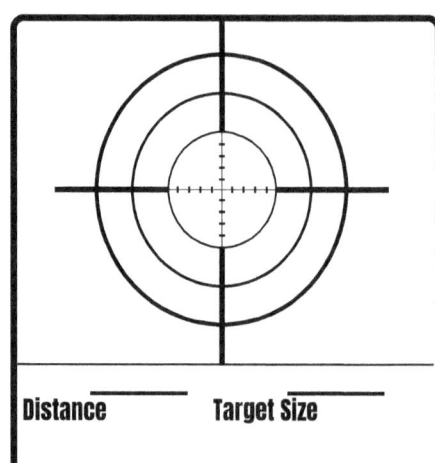

Distance _____ Target Size _____

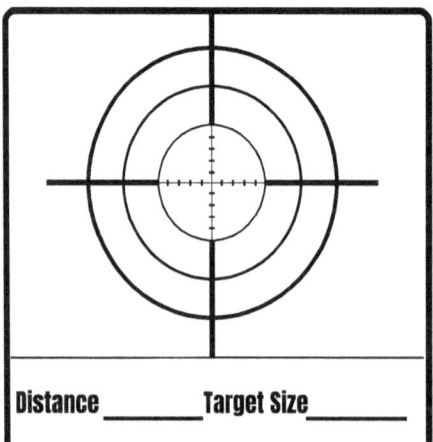

Distance _____ Target Size _____

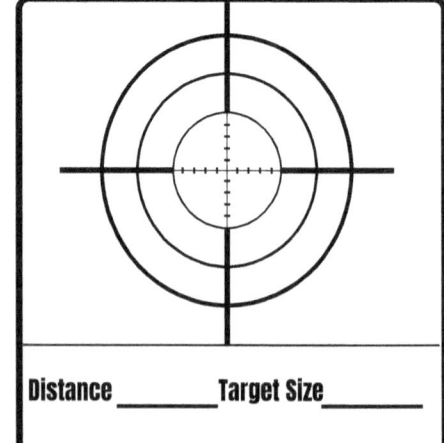

Distance _____ Target Size _____

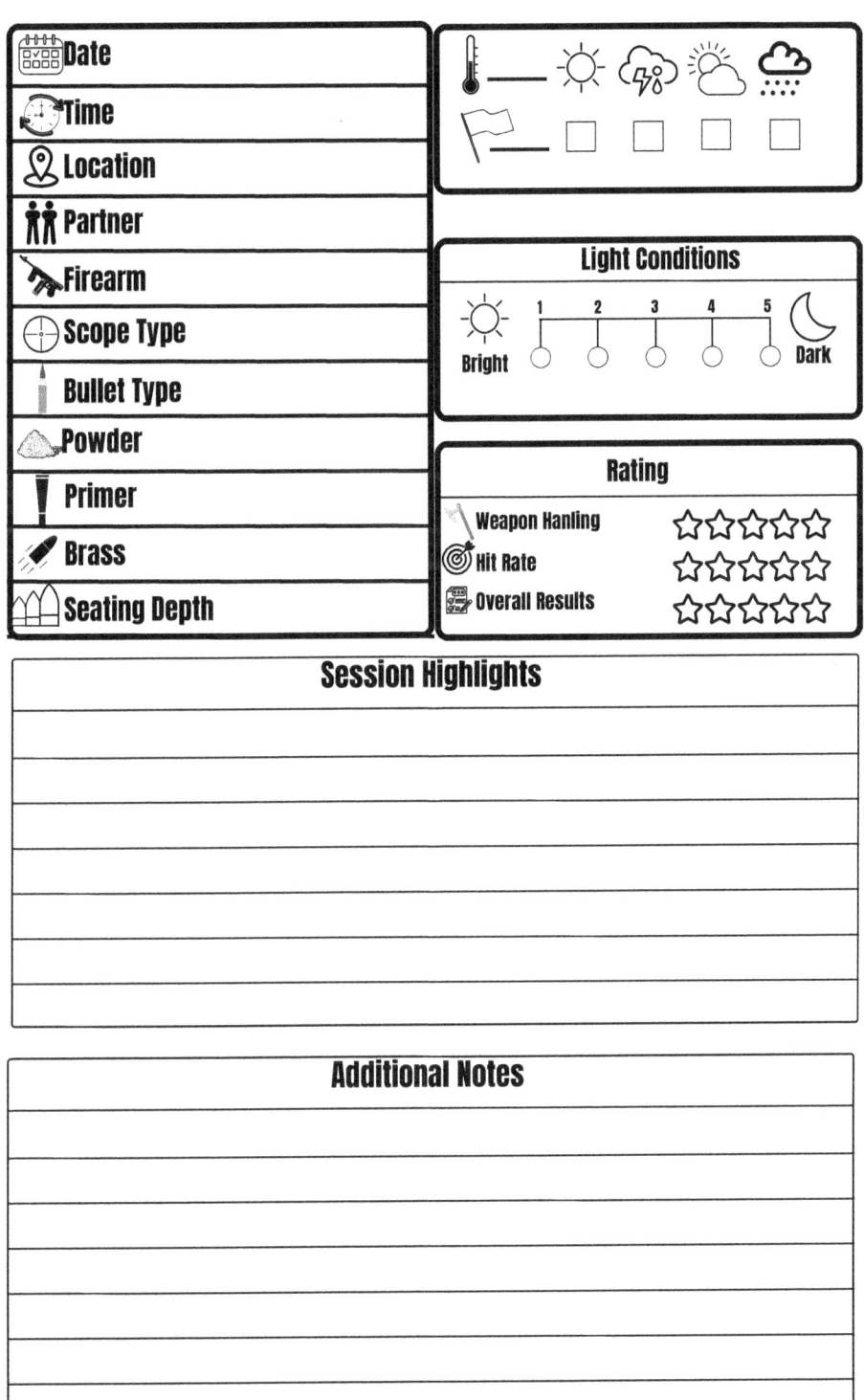

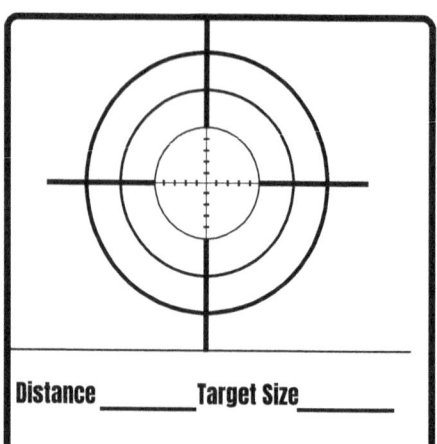
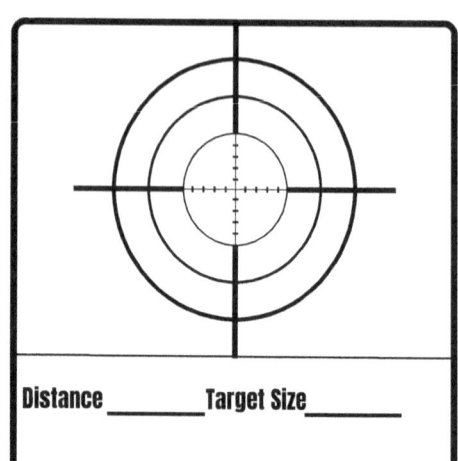
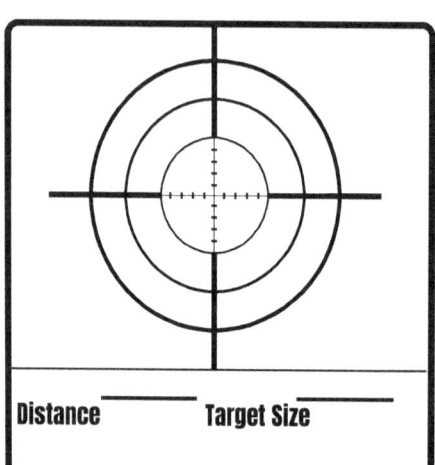
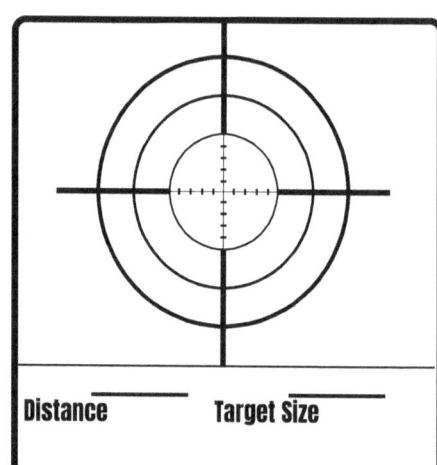
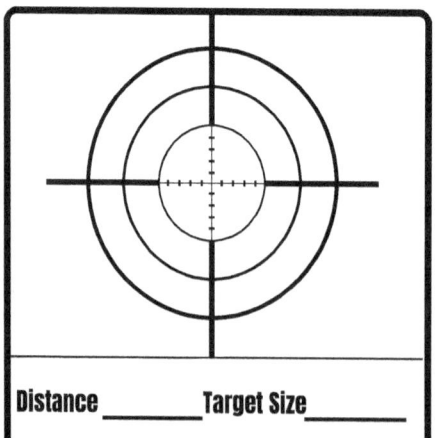
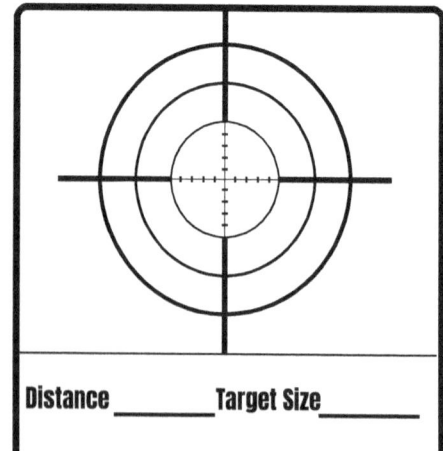

📅 Date	
🕐 Time	
📍 Location	
👥 Partner	
🔫 Firearm	
🔭 Scope Type	
Bullet Type	
Powder	
Primer	
Brass	
Seating Depth	

🌡️ ——— ☀️ ⛈️ ⛅ 🌧️
🚩 ——— ☐ ☐ ☐ ☐

Light Conditions

Bright 1 2 3 4 5 Dark

Rating

Weapon Hanling	☆☆☆☆☆
Hit Rate	☆☆☆☆☆
Overall Results	☆☆☆☆☆

Session Highlights

_____
_____
_____
_____
_____
_____
_____
_____
_____

Additional Notes

_____
_____
_____
_____
_____
_____
_____
_____

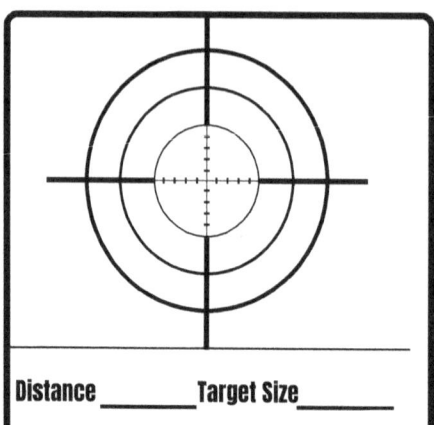
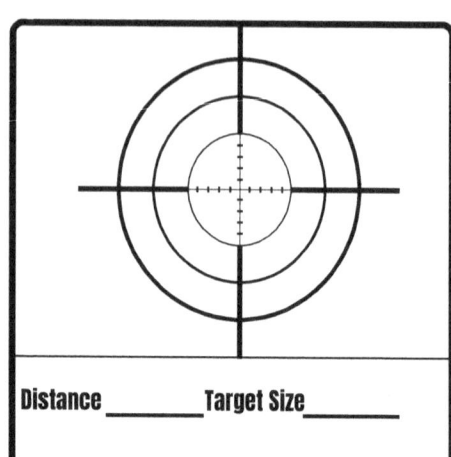
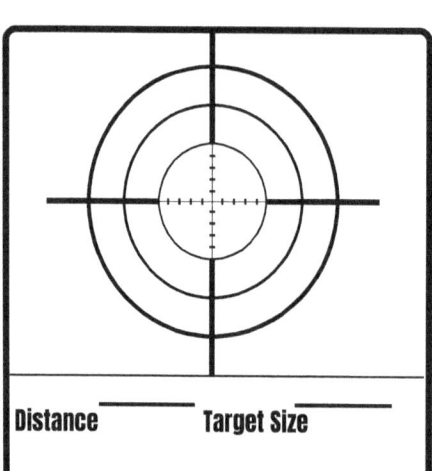
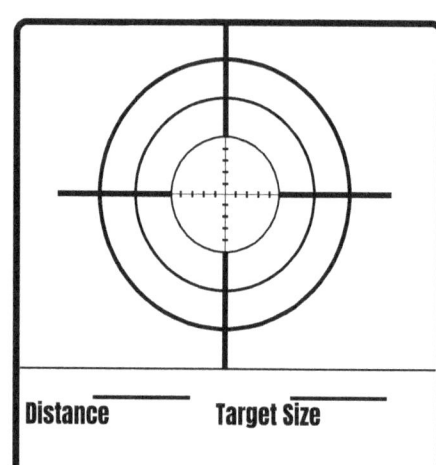
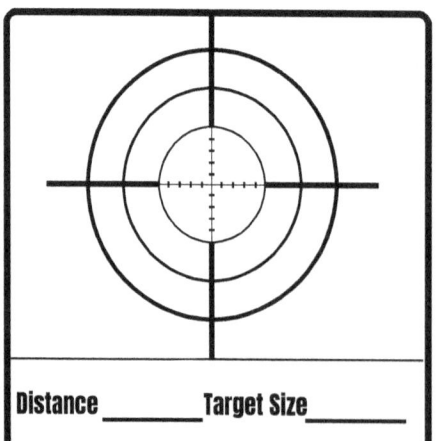
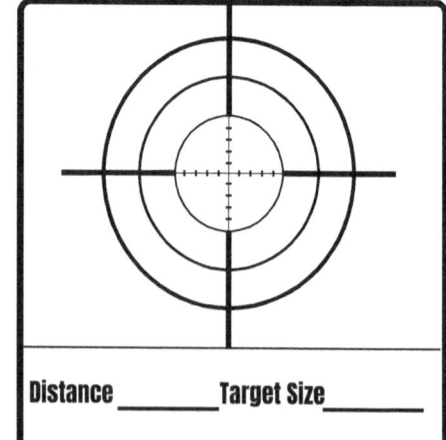

Date	
Time	
Location	
Partner	
Firearm	
Scope Type	
Bullet Type	
Powder	
Primer	
Brass	
Seating Depth	

Light Conditions
Bright 1 — 2 — 3 — 4 — 5 Dark

Rating
- Weapon Hanling ☆☆☆☆☆
- Hit Rate ☆☆☆☆☆
- Overall Results ☆☆☆☆☆

Session Highlights

Additional Notes

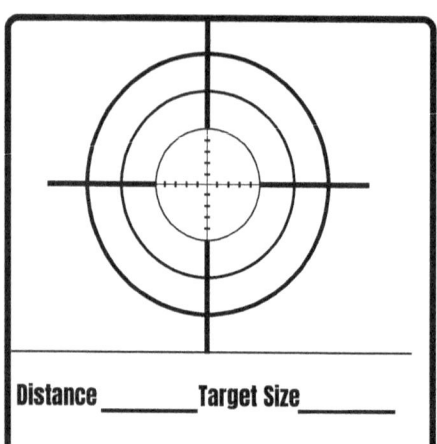

Distance _____ Target Size _____

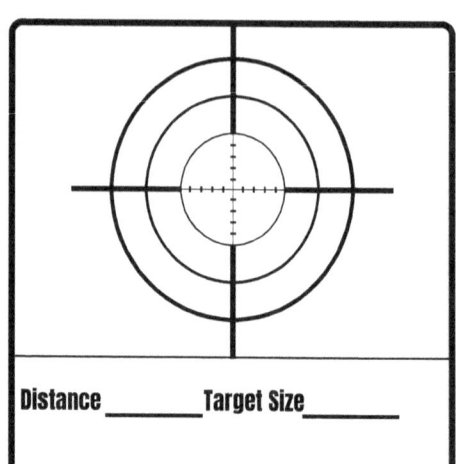

Distance _____ Target Size _____

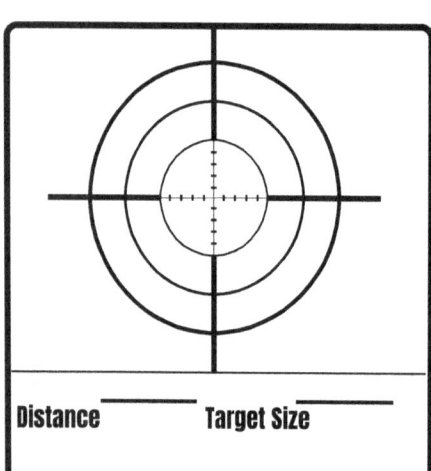

Distance _____ Target Size _____

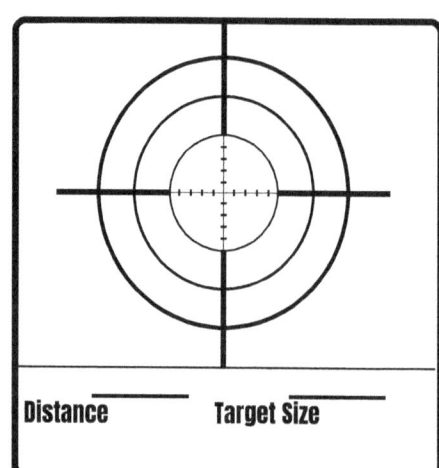

Distance _____ Target Size _____

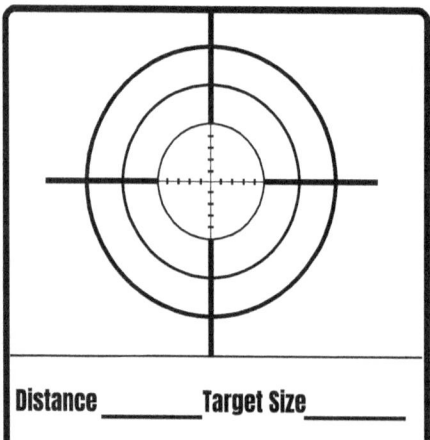

Distance _____ Target Size _____

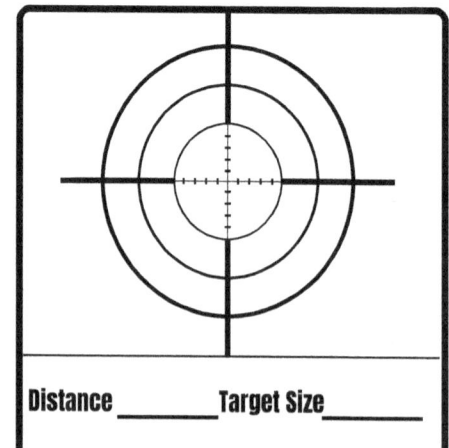

Distance _____ Target Size _____

📅 Date	
⏱ Time	
📍 Location	
👥 Partner	
🔫 Firearm	
🔭 Scope Type	
🔹 Bullet Type	
🔺 Powder	
❗ Primer	
🚀 Brass	
🔻 Seating Depth	

Weather: 🌡 ____ ☀ ⛈ 🌤 🌨
🚩 ____ ☐ ☐ ☐ ☐

Light Conditions
Bright ☀ 1○ 2○ 3○ 4○ 5○ 🌙 Dark

Rating
- Weapon Hanling ☆☆☆☆☆
- Hit Rate ☆☆☆☆☆
- Overall Results ☆☆☆☆☆

Session Highlights

_____
_____
_____
_____
_____
_____
_____
_____
_____

Additional Notes

_____
_____
_____
_____
_____
_____
_____
_____

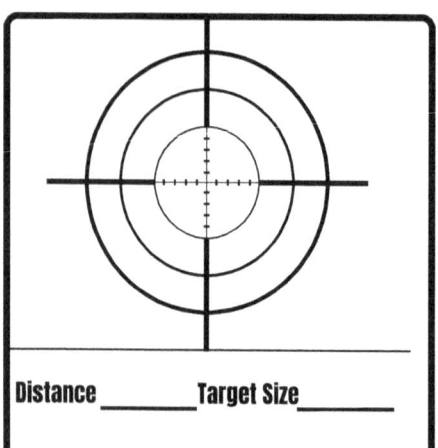

Distance _____ Target Size _____

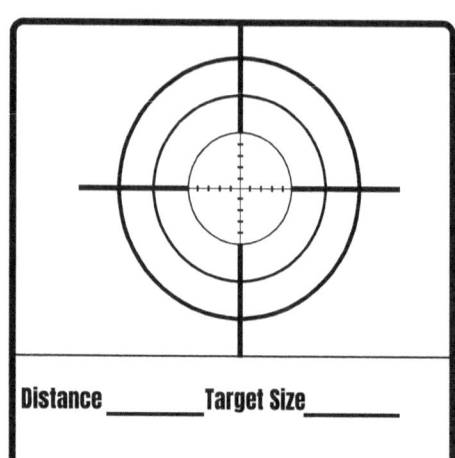

Distance _____ Target Size _____

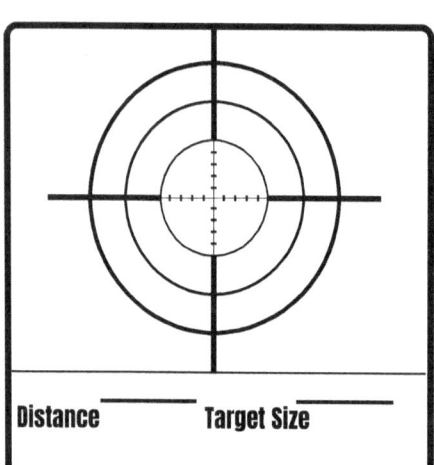

Distance _____ Target Size _____

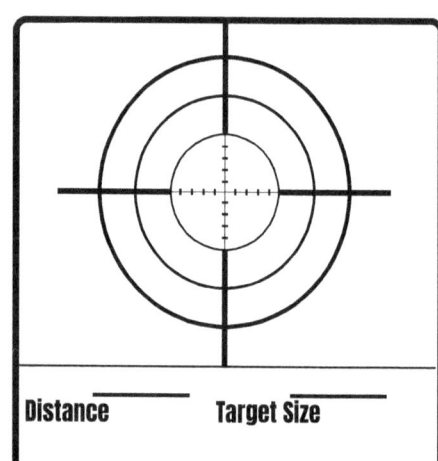

Distance _____ Target Size _____

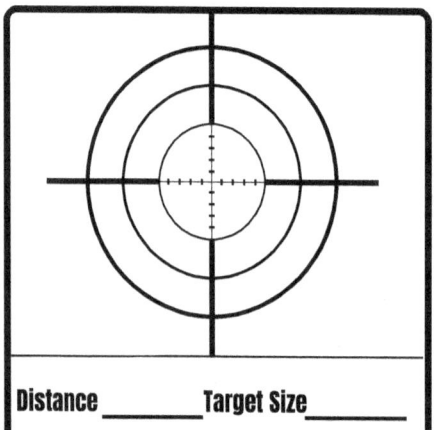

Distance _____ Target Size _____

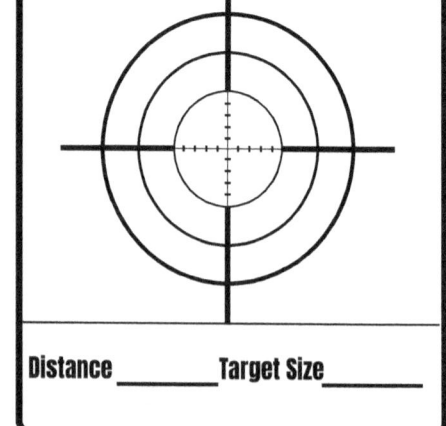

Distance _____ Target Size _____

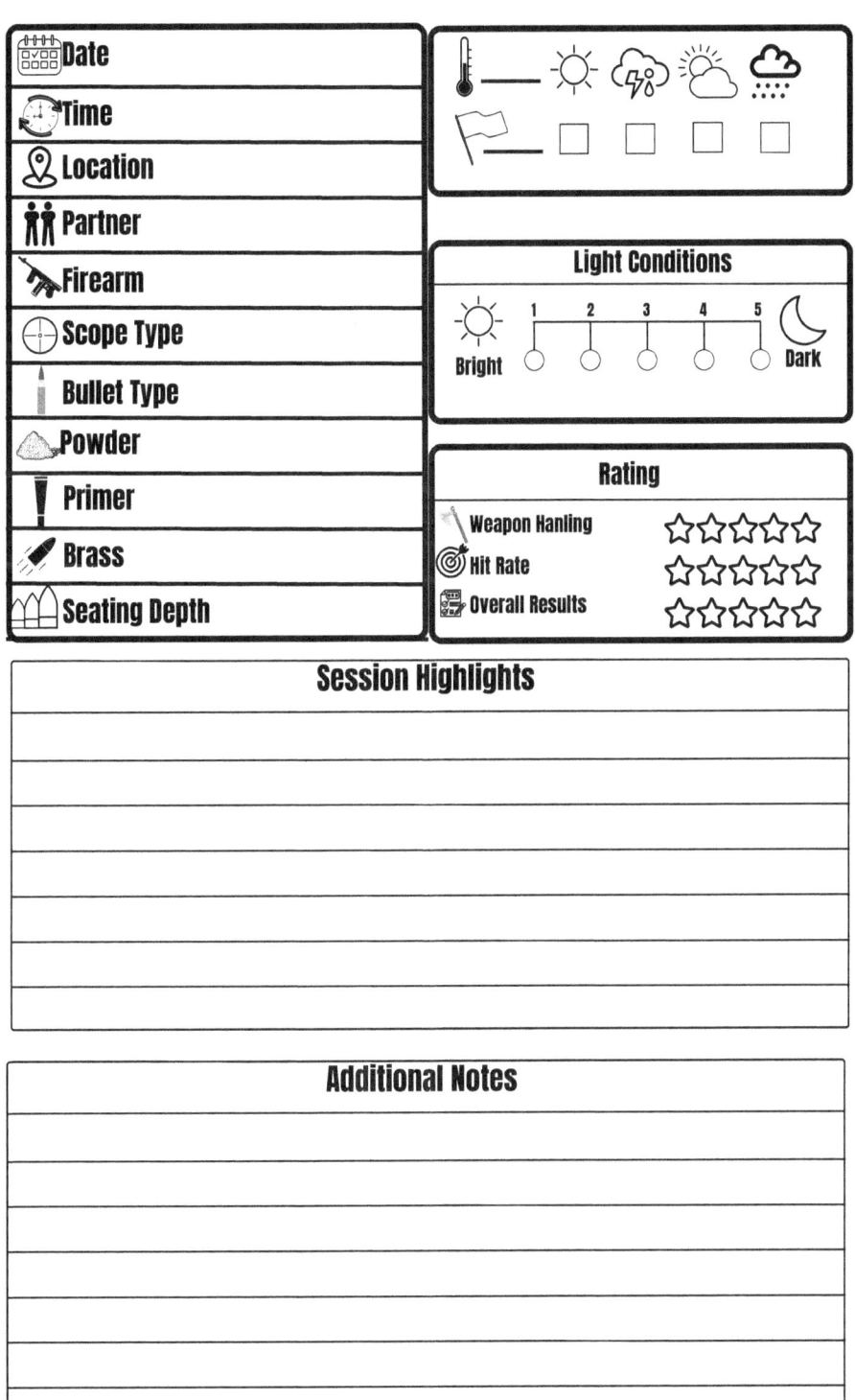

Date	
Time	
Location	
Partner	
Firearm	
Scope Type	
Bullet Type	
Powder	
Primer	
Brass	
Seating Depth	

Light Conditions

Bright 1 2 3 4 5 Dark

Rating

- Weapon Hanling ☆☆☆☆☆
- Hit Rate ☆☆☆☆☆
- Overall Results ☆☆☆☆☆

Session Highlights

Additional Notes

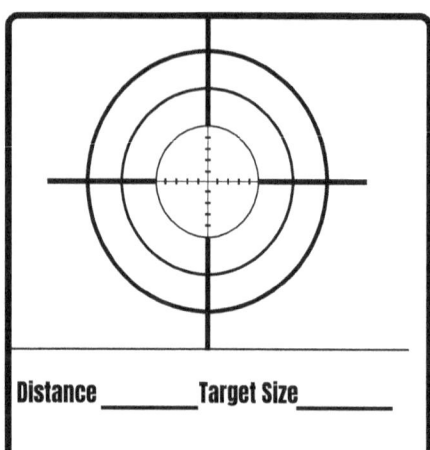
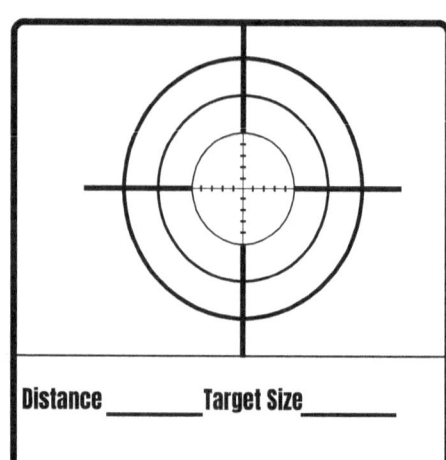
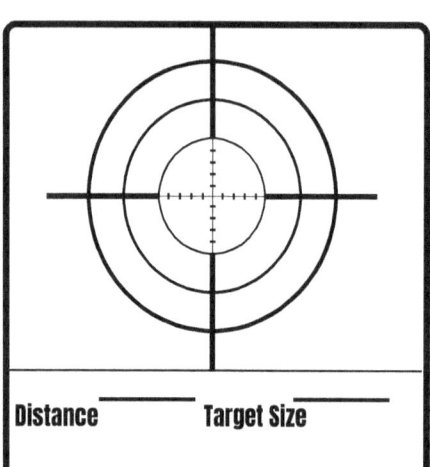
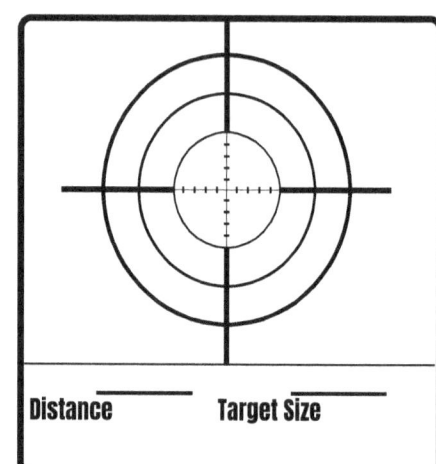
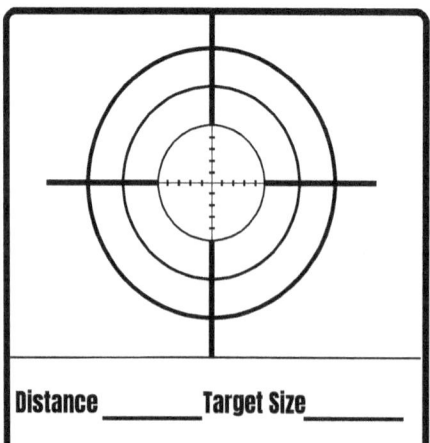
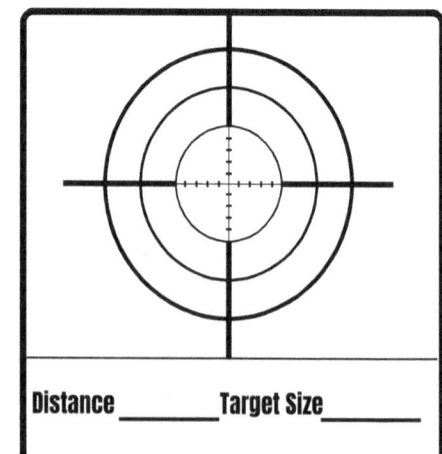

📅 Date	
⏱ Time	
📍 Location	
👥 Partner	
🔫 Firearm	
🎯 Scope Type	
🔸 Bullet Type	
🔺 Powder	
🔻 Primer	
🚀 Brass	
🔺 Seating Depth	

🌡 ─── ☀ ⛈ 🌤 🌨
🚩 ─── ☐ ☐ ☐ ☐

Light Conditions

☀ 1 — 2 — 3 — 4 — 5 🌙
Bright ○ ○ ○ ○ ○ Dark

Rating

Weapon Hanling	☆☆☆☆☆
Hit Rate	☆☆☆☆☆
Overall Results	☆☆☆☆☆

Session Highlights

Additional Notes

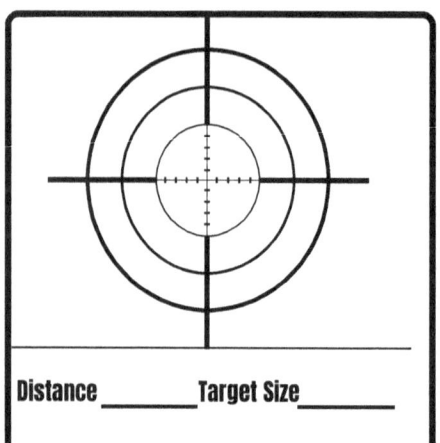
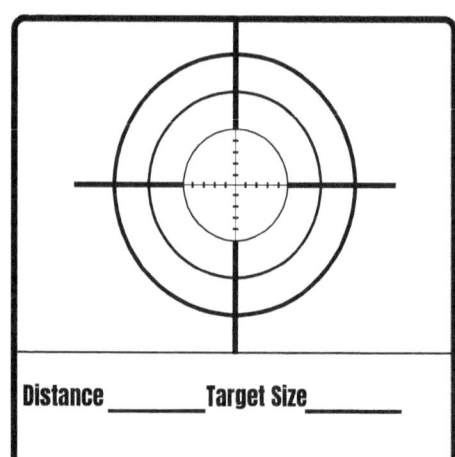
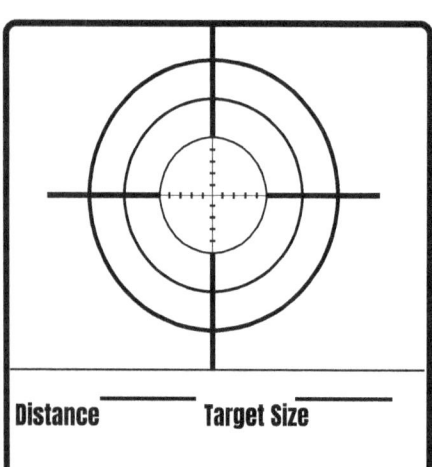
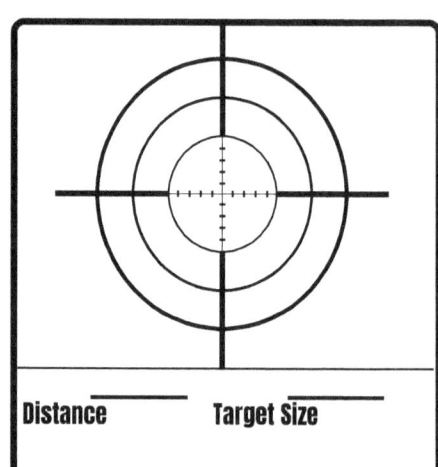
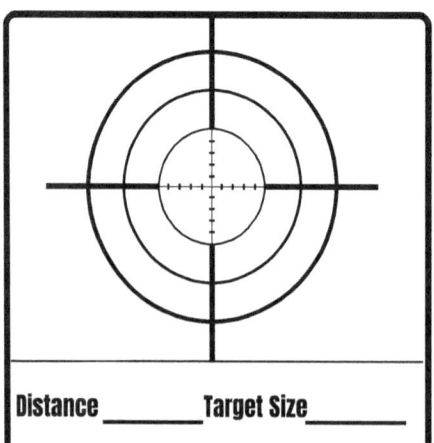
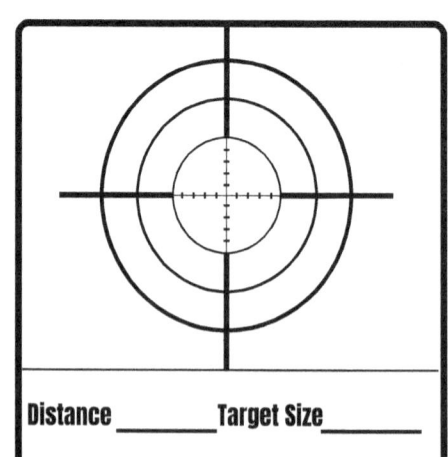

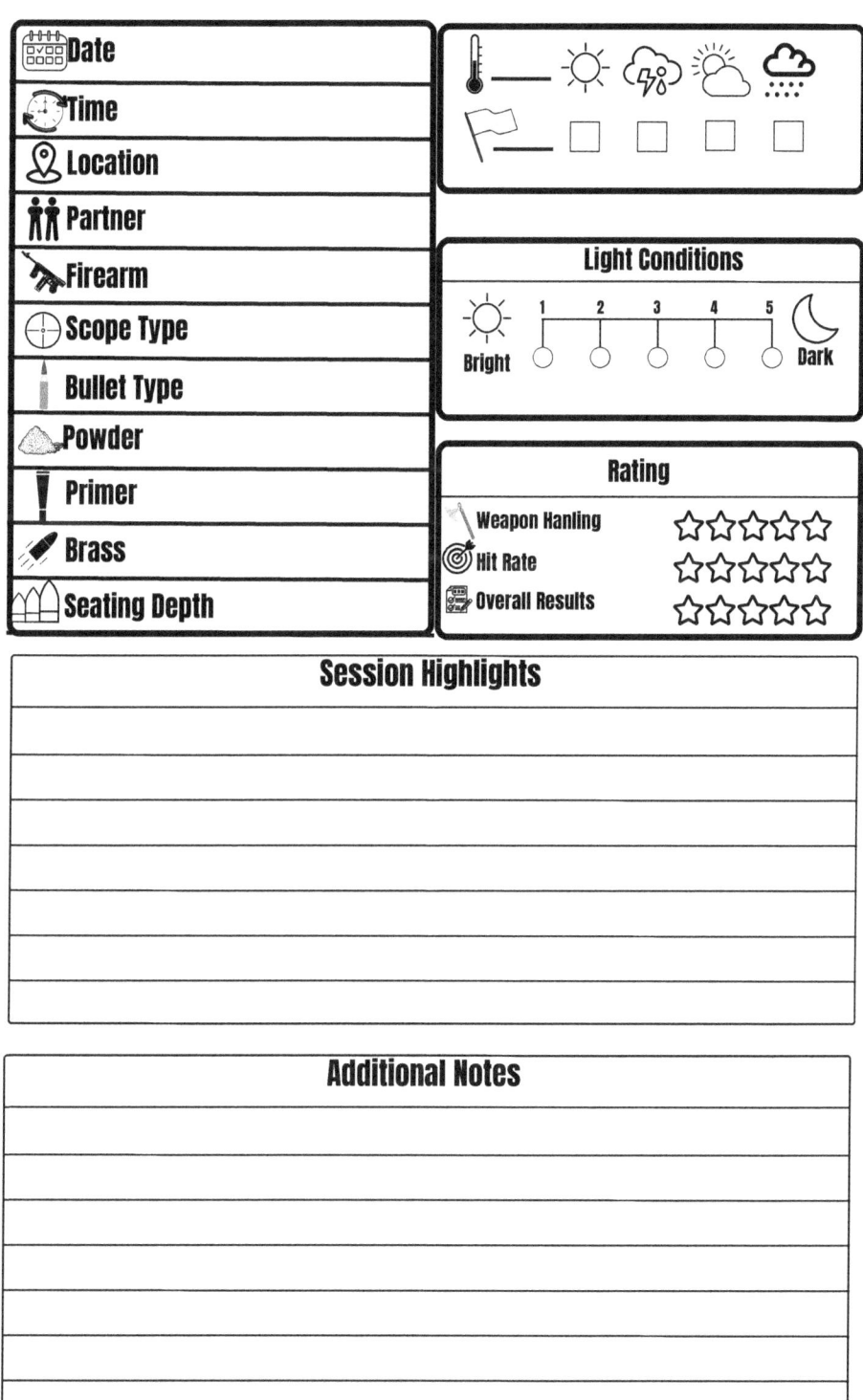

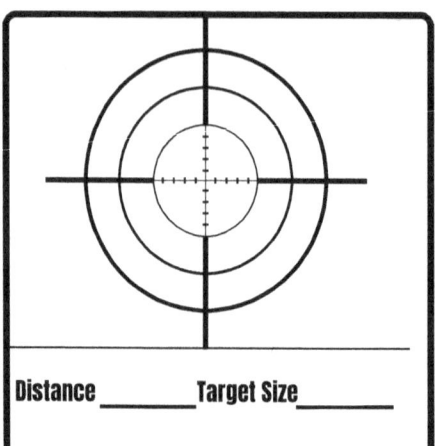
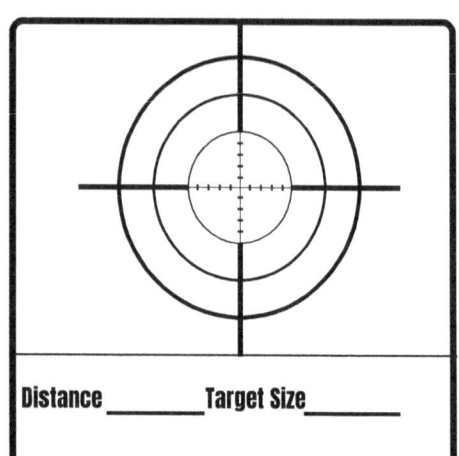
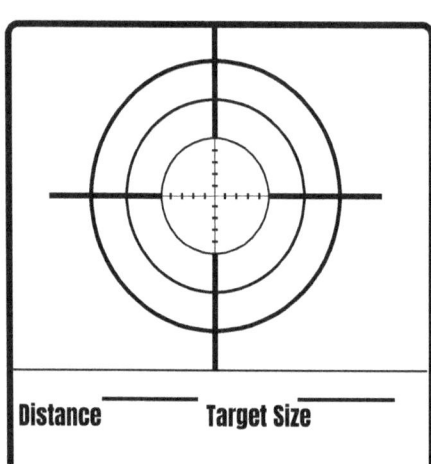
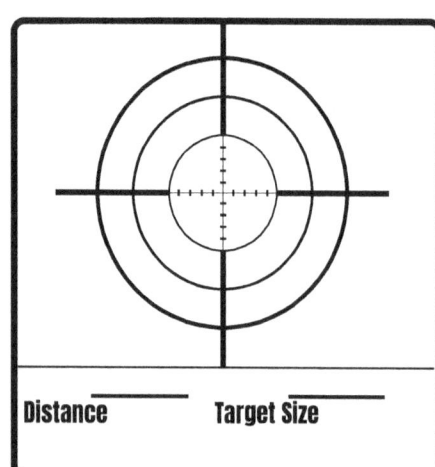
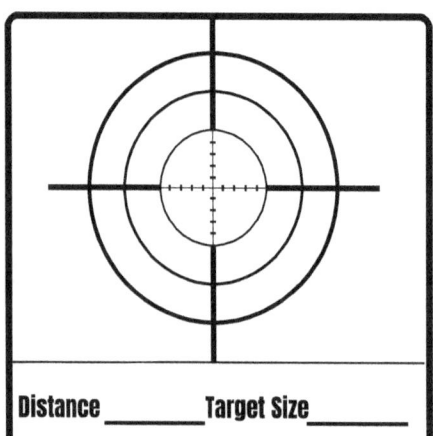
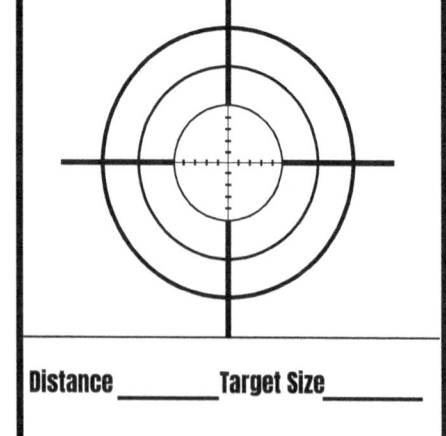

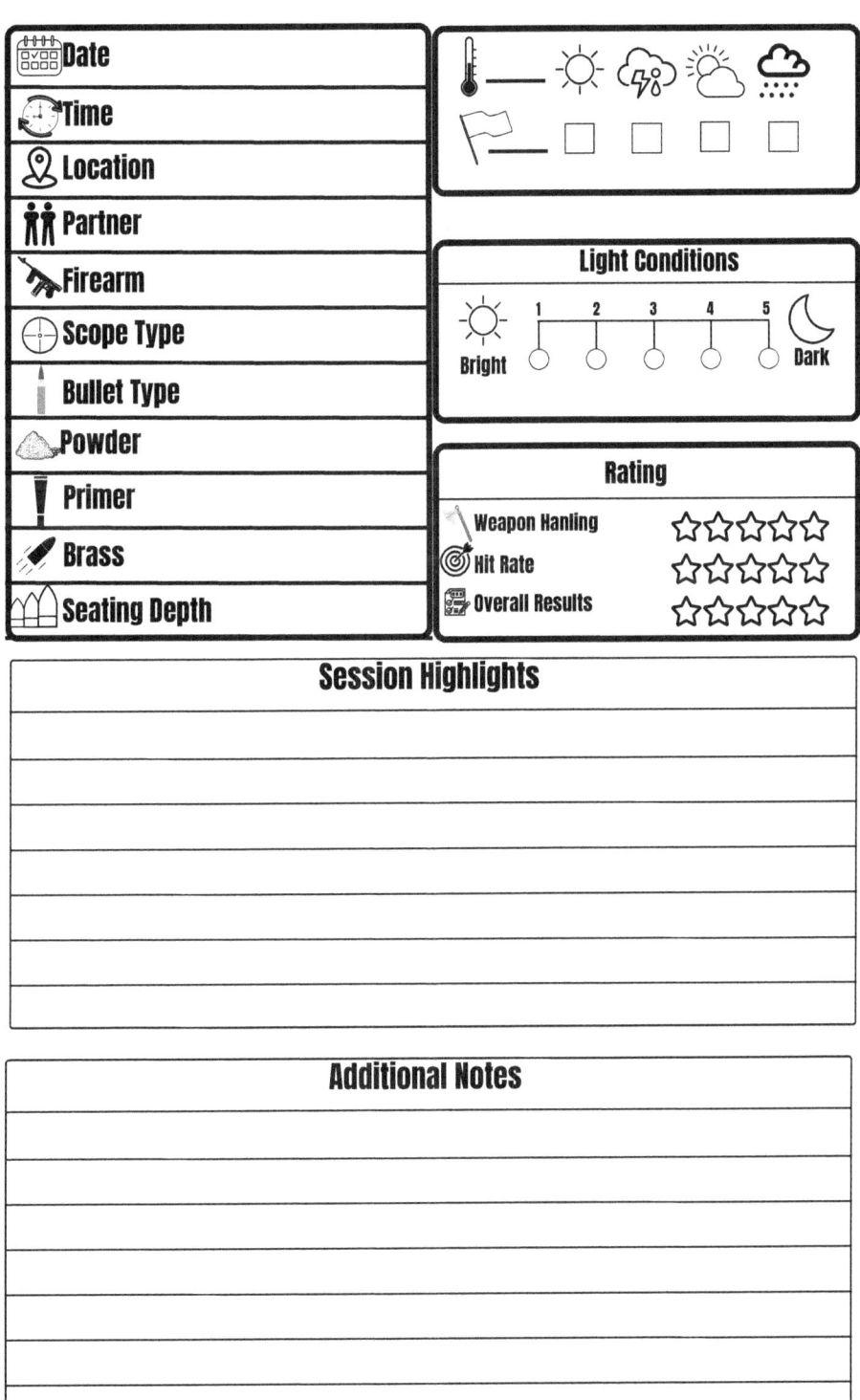

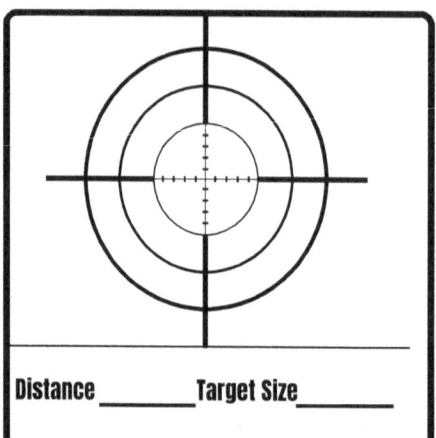

Distance _____ Target Size _____

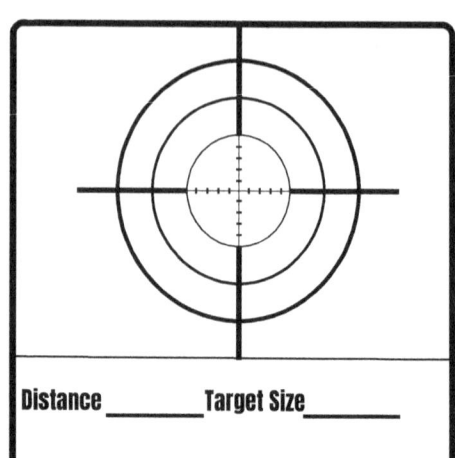

Distance _____ Target Size _____

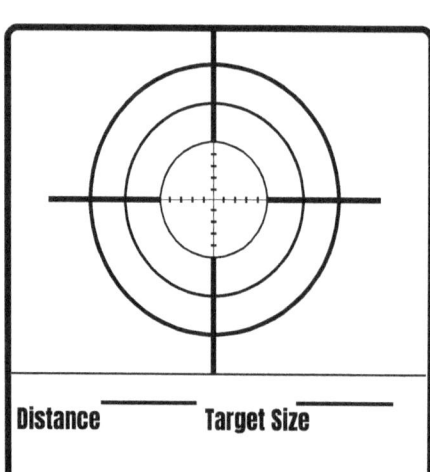

Distance _____ Target Size _____

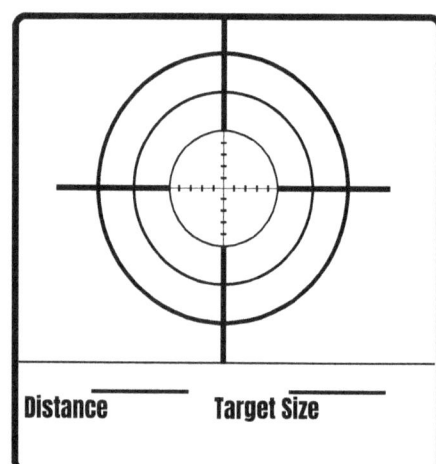

Distance _____ Target Size _____

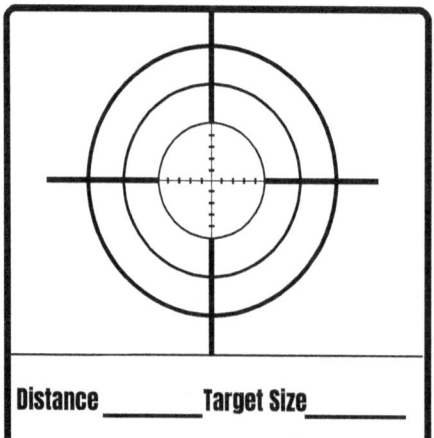

Distance _____ Target Size _____

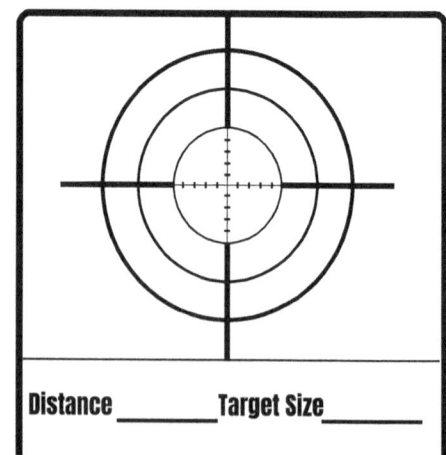

Distance _____ Target Size _____

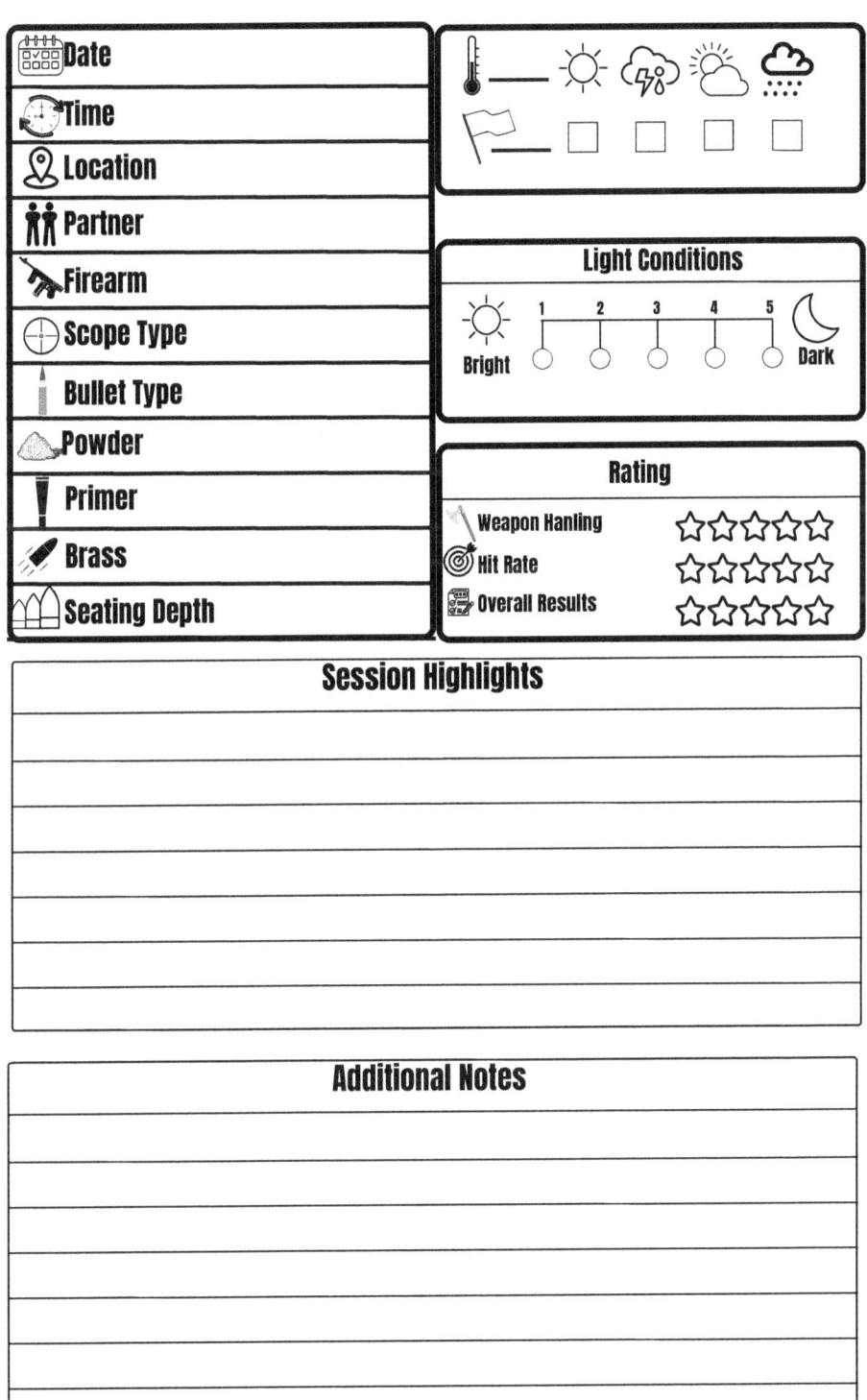

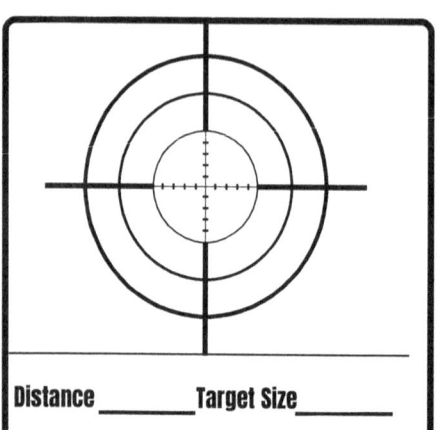
Distance _____ Target Size _____

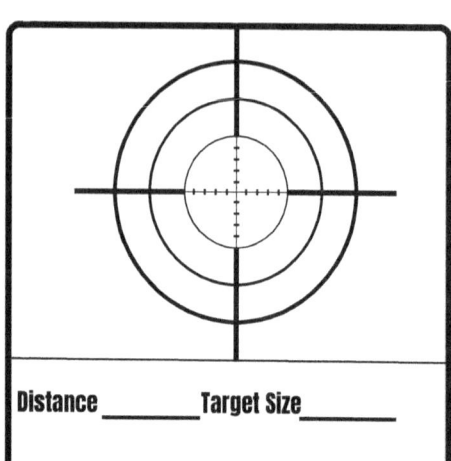
Distance _____ Target Size _____

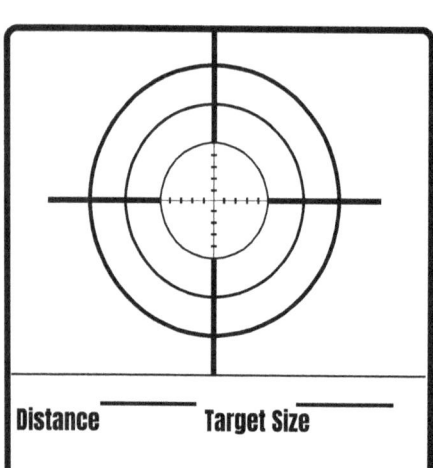
Distance _____ Target Size _____

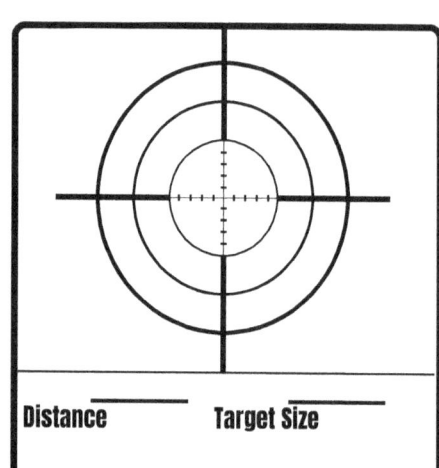
Distance _____ Target Size _____

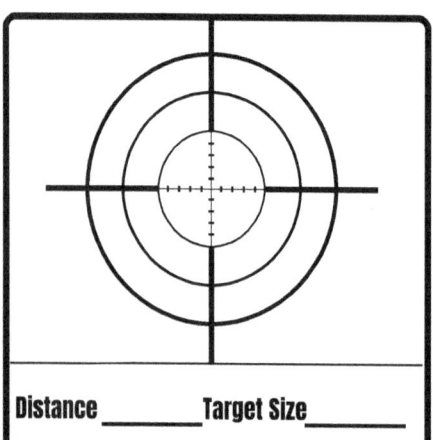
Distance _____ Target Size _____

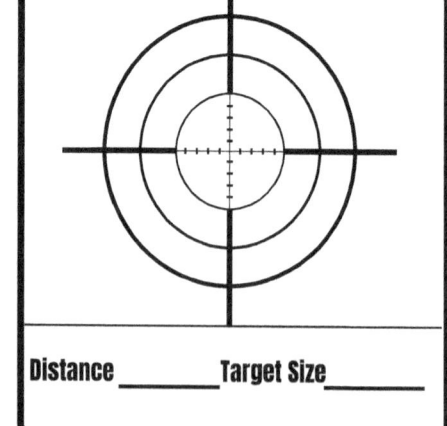
Distance _____ Target Size _____

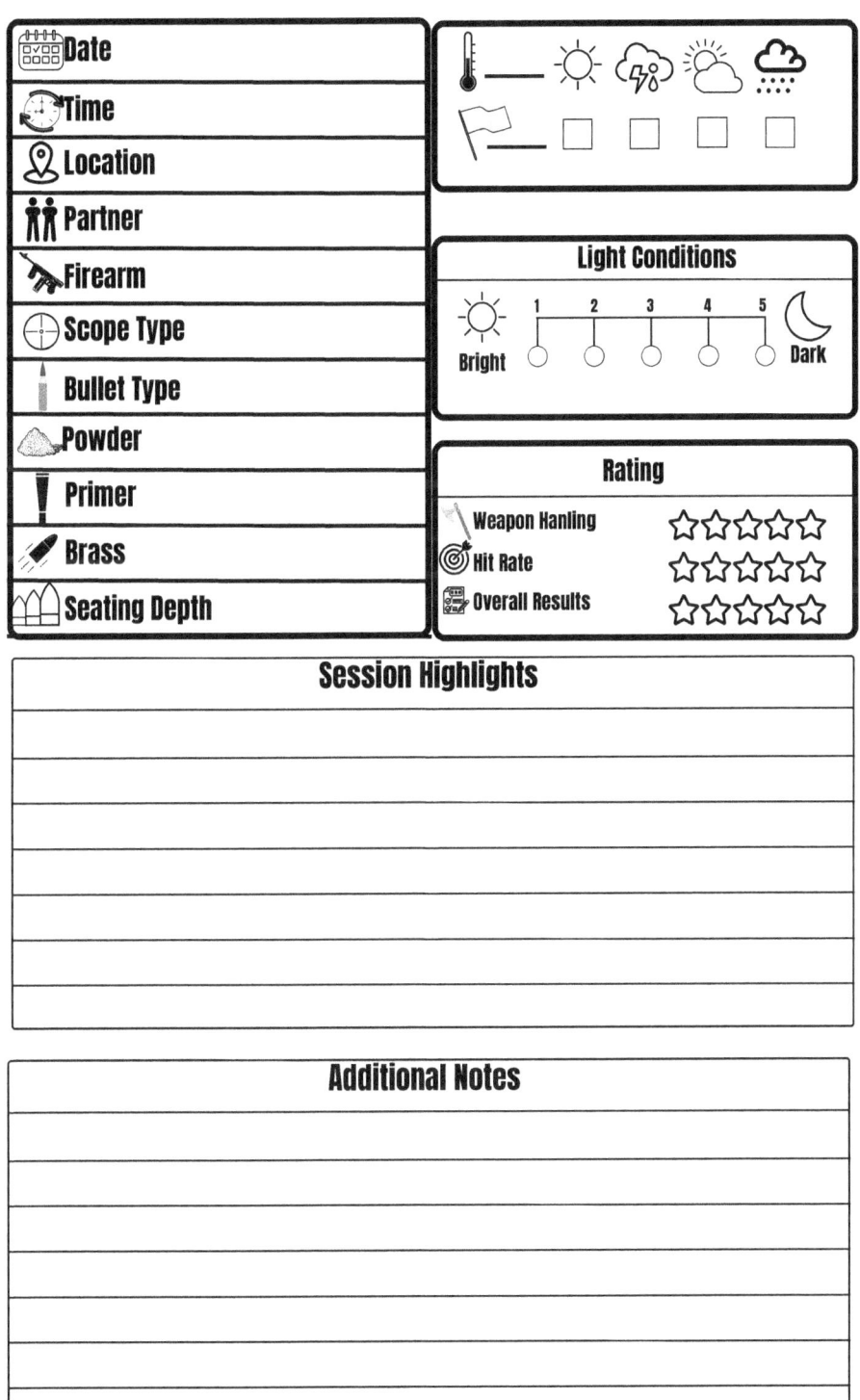

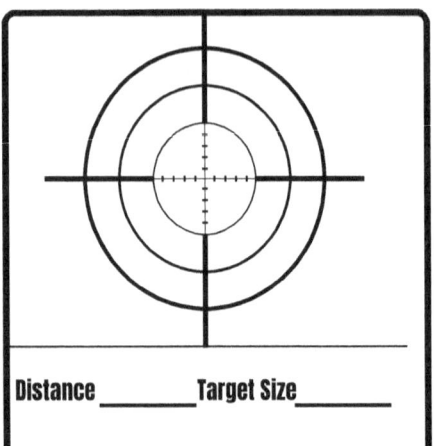
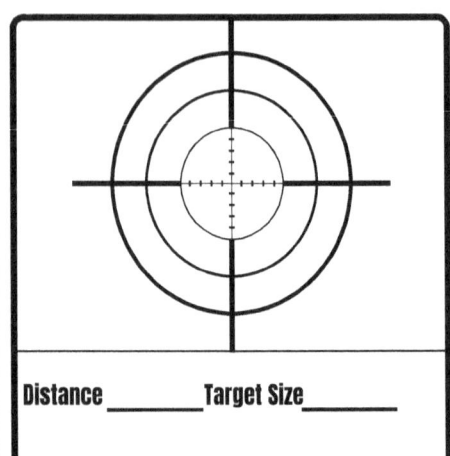
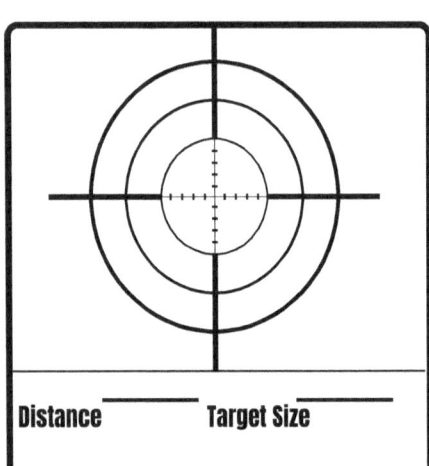
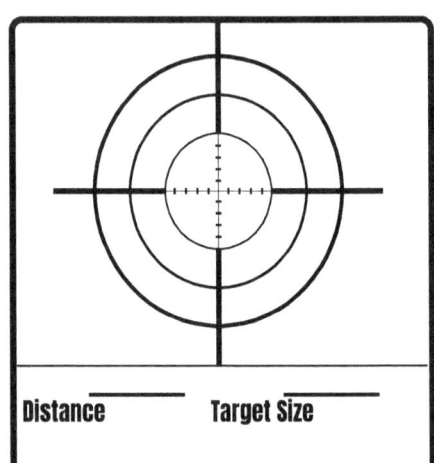
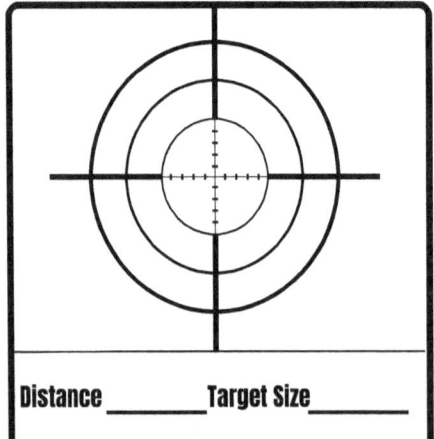
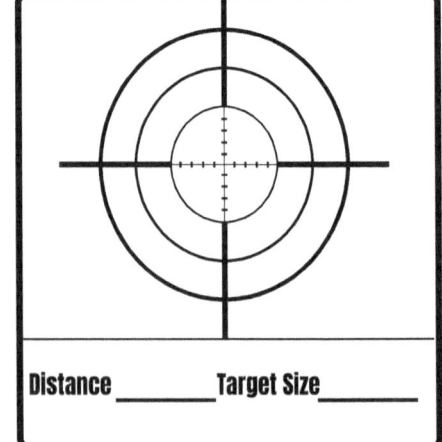

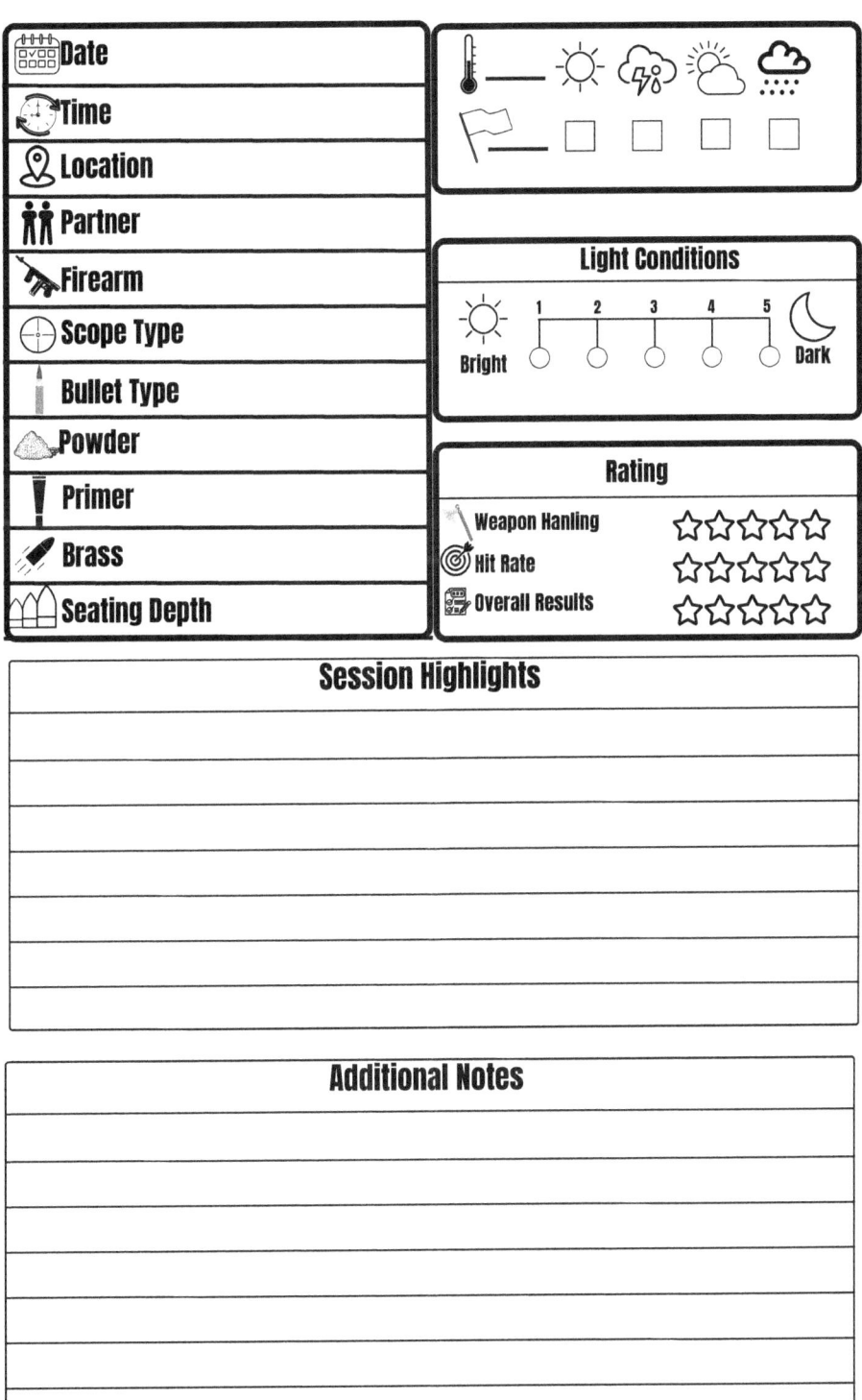

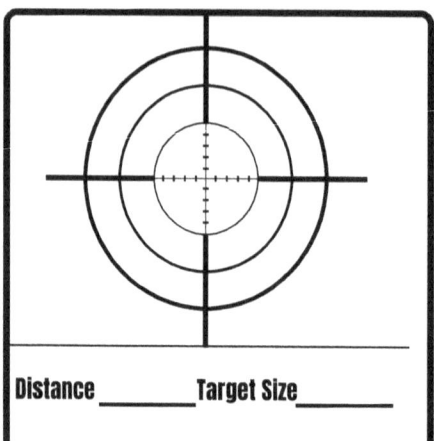
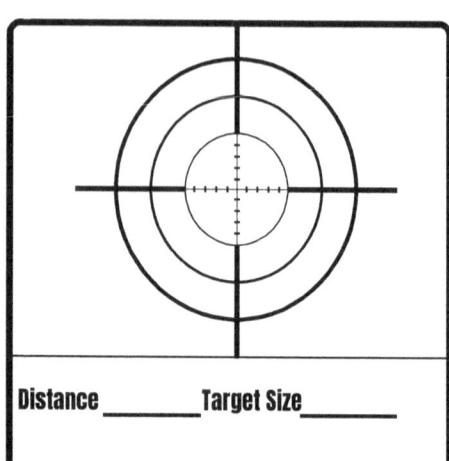
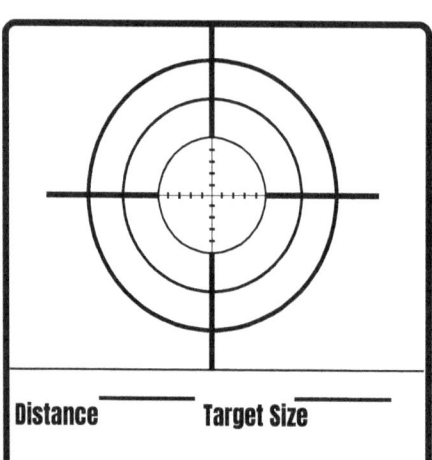
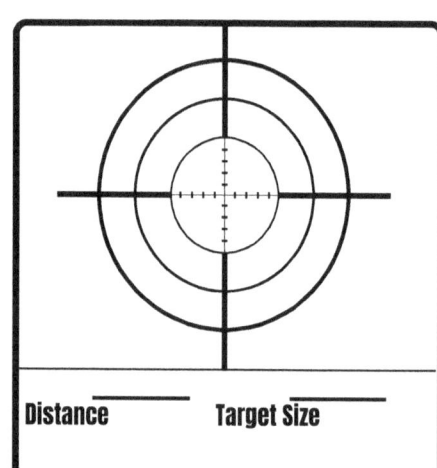
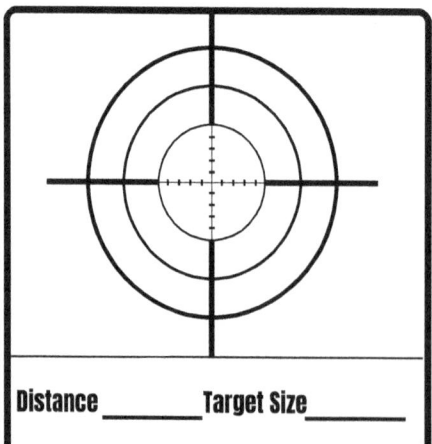
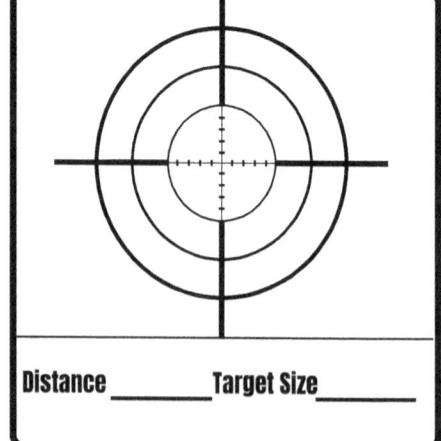

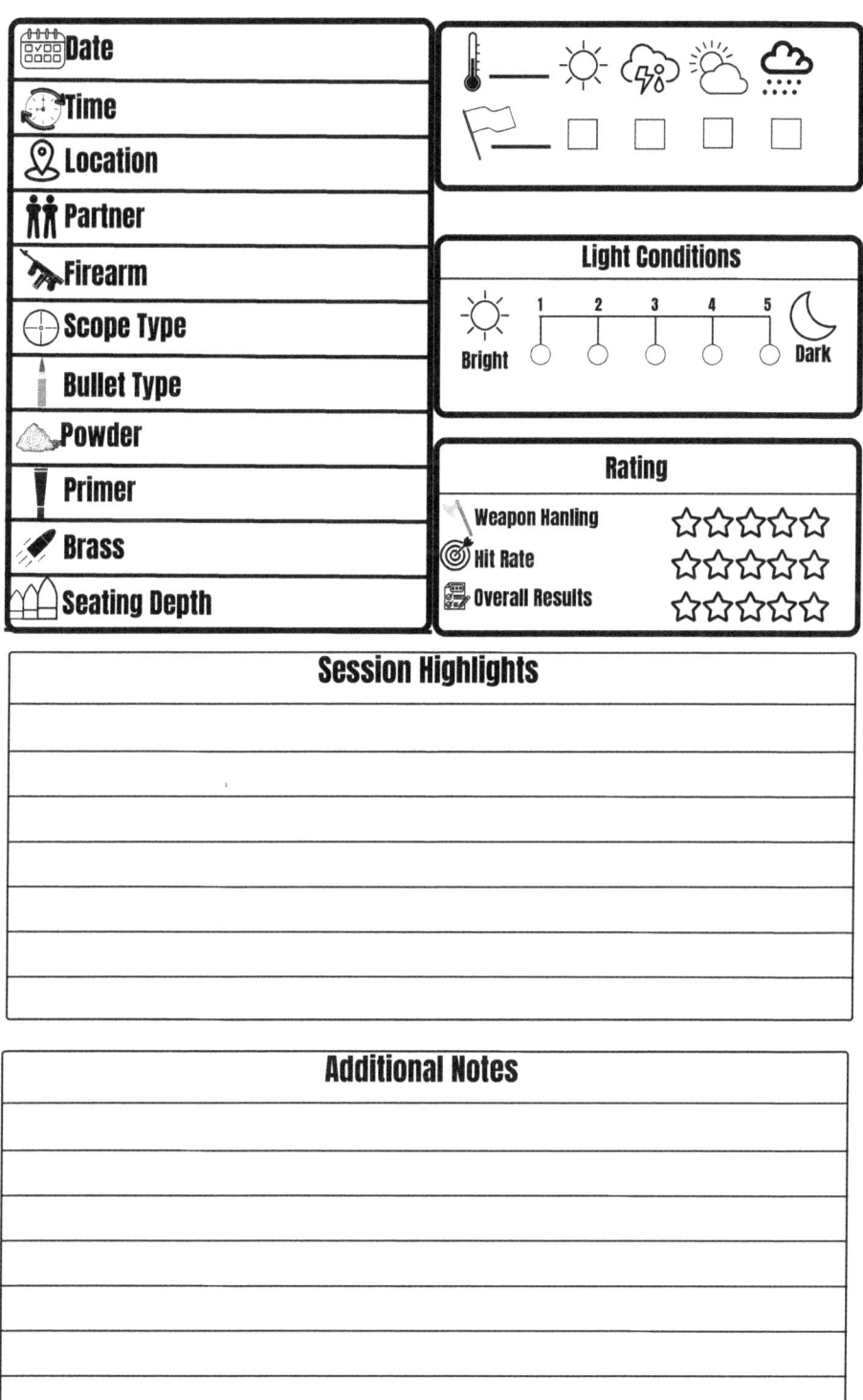

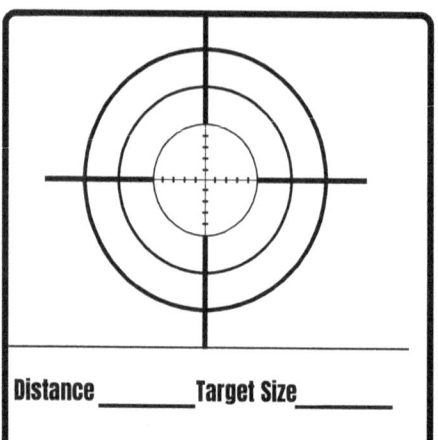

Distance _____ Target Size _____

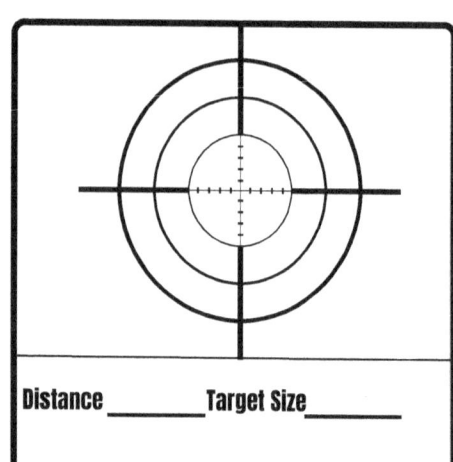

Distance _____ Target Size _____

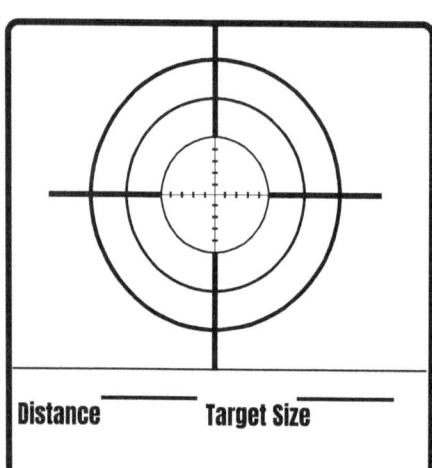

Distance _____ Target Size _____

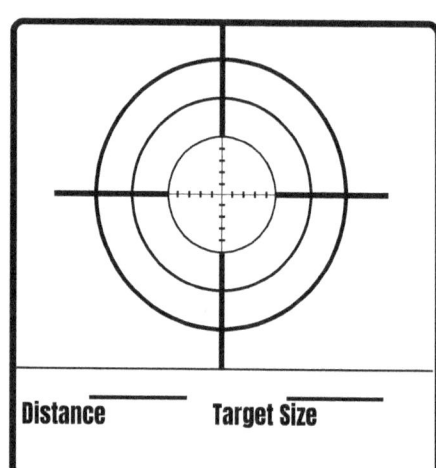

Distance _____ Target Size _____

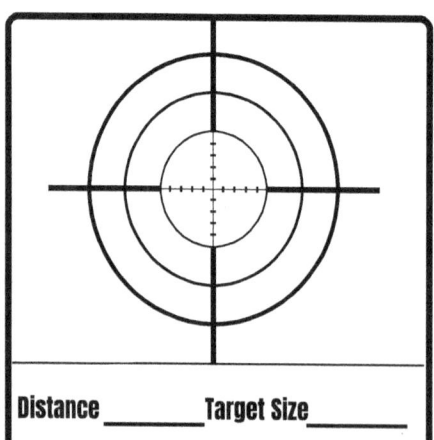

Distance _____ Target Size _____

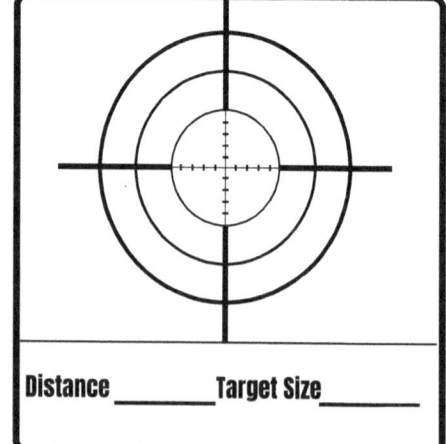

Distance _____ Target Size _____

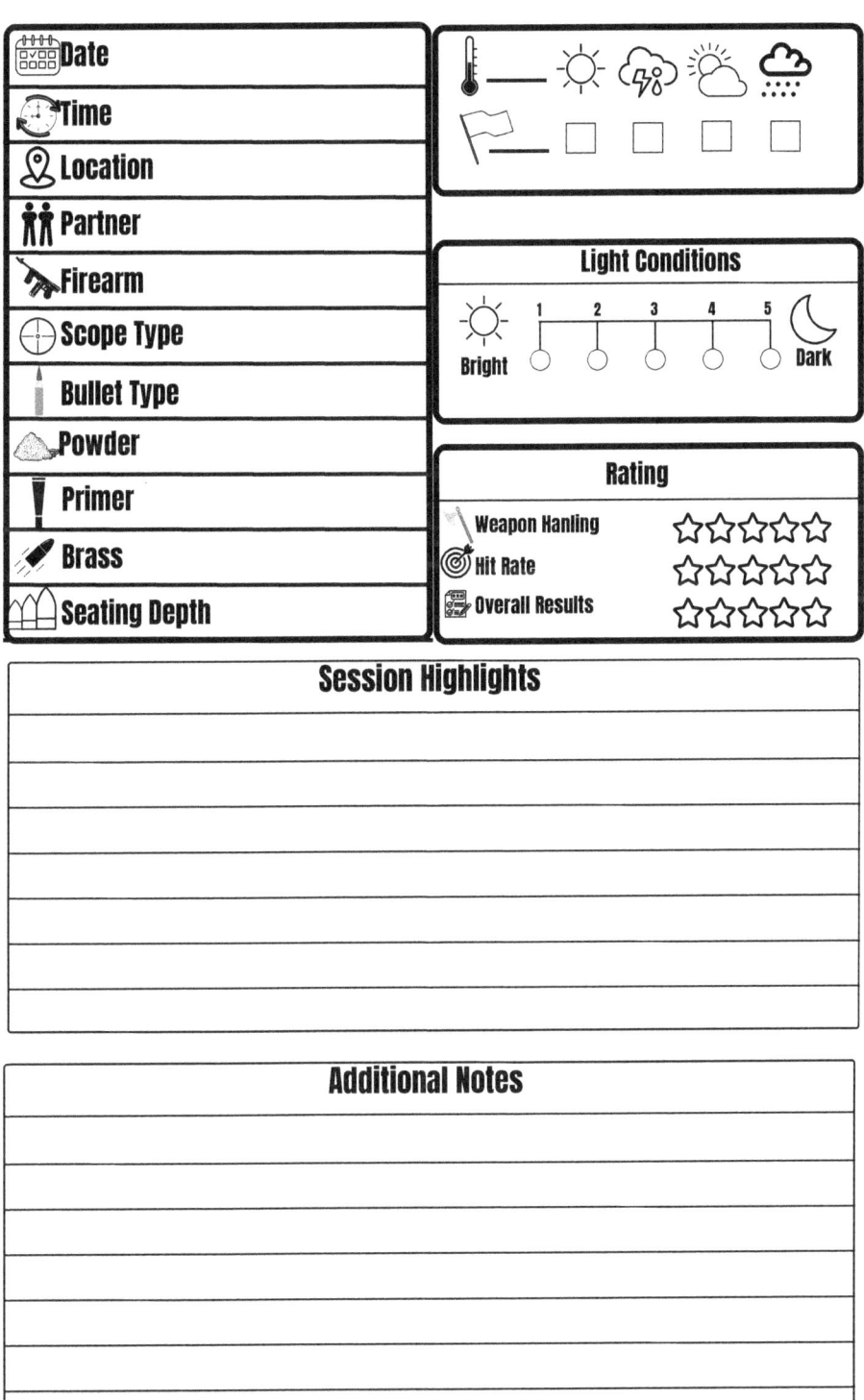

Date	
Time	
Location	
Partner	
Firearm	
Scope Type	
Bullet Type	
Powder	
Primer	
Brass	
Seating Depth	

Light Conditions

Bright 1 — 2 — 3 — 4 — 5 Dark

Rating

Weapon Hanling	☆☆☆☆☆
Hit Rate	☆☆☆☆☆
Overall Results	☆☆☆☆☆

Session Highlights

Additional Notes

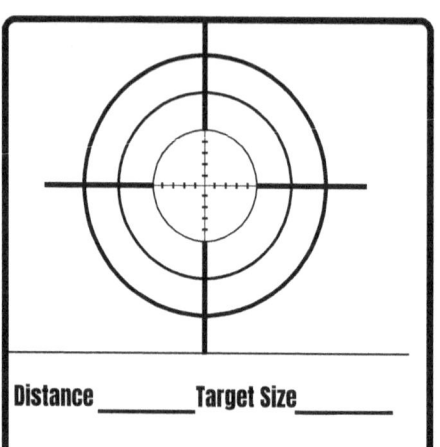

Distance _____ Target Size _____

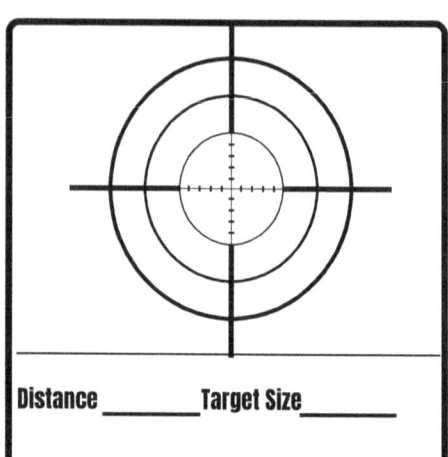

Distance _____ Target Size _____

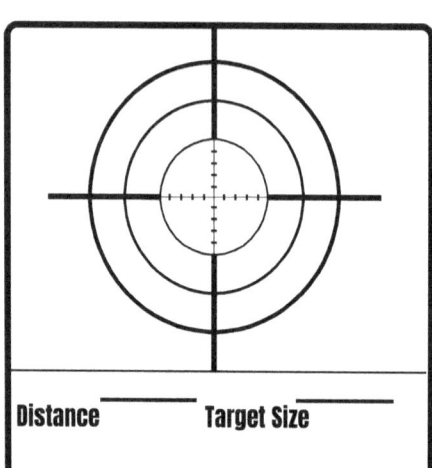

Distance _____ Target Size _____

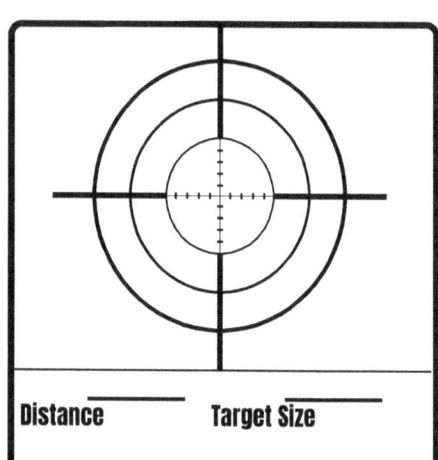

Distance _____ Target Size _____

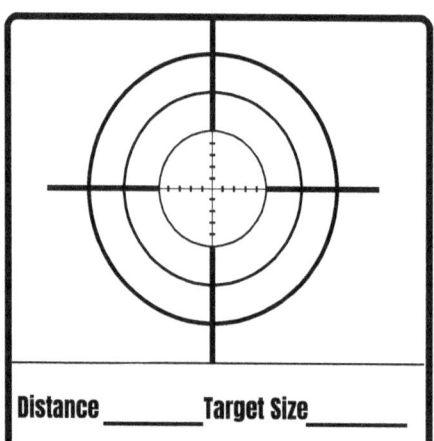

Distance _____ Target Size _____

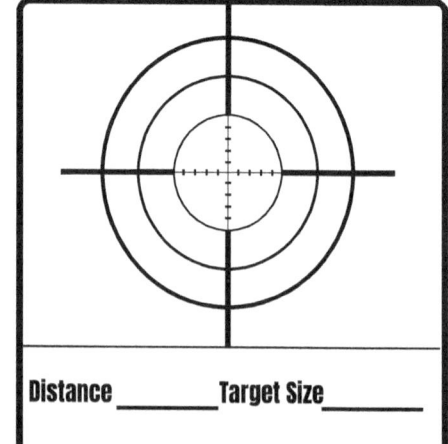

Distance _____ Target Size _____

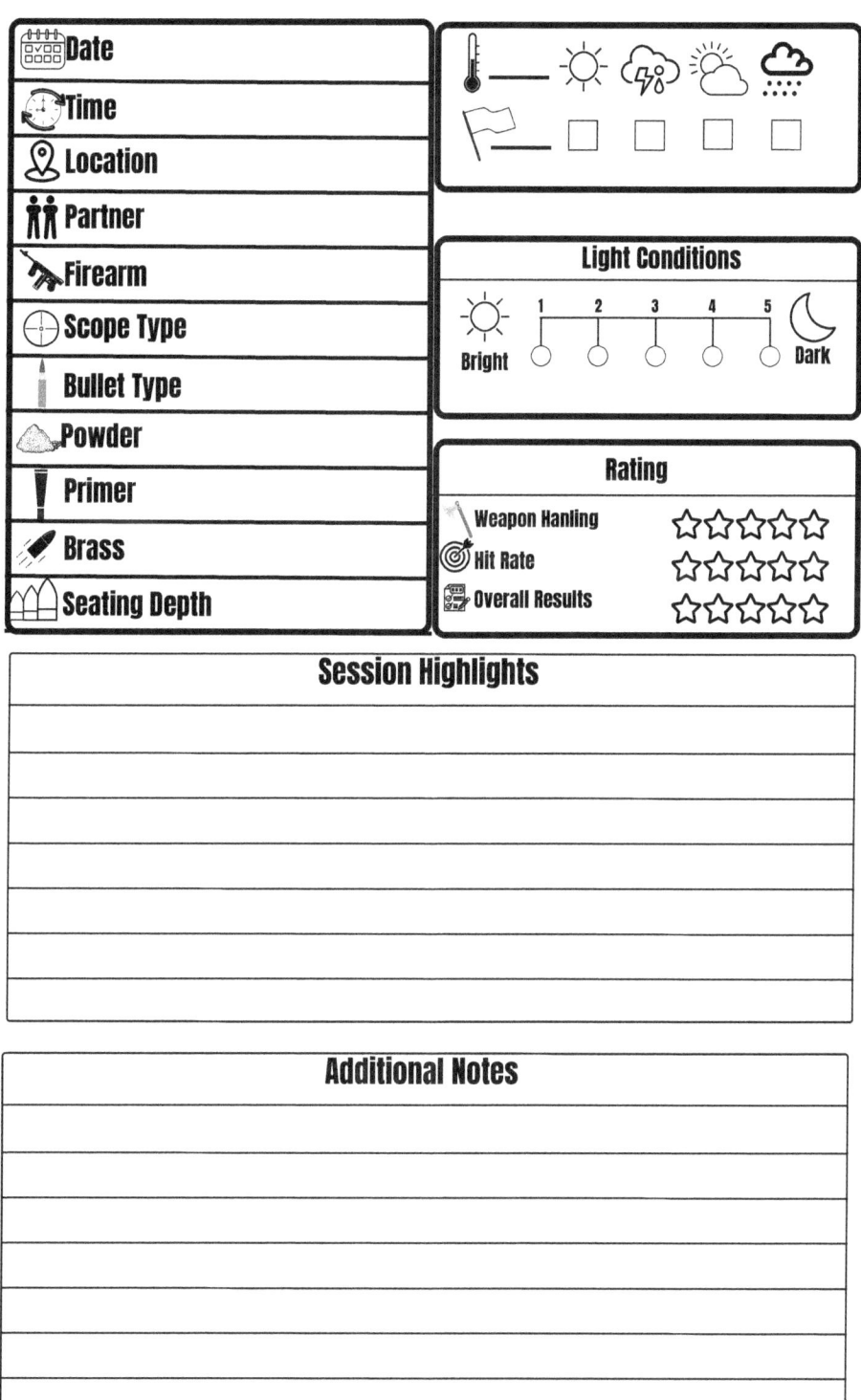

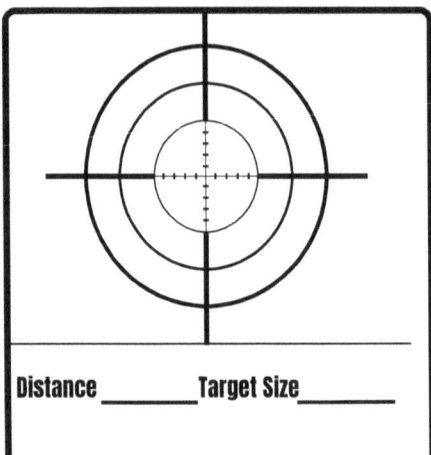

Distance _____ Target Size _____

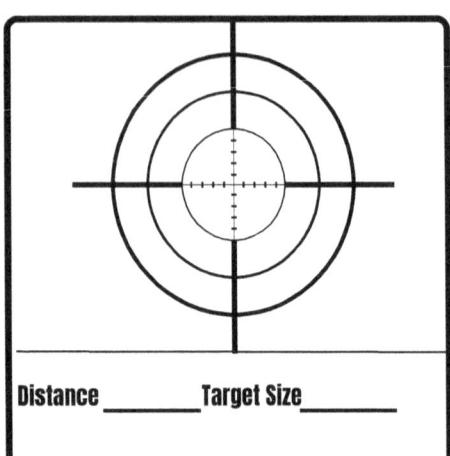

Distance _____ Target Size _____

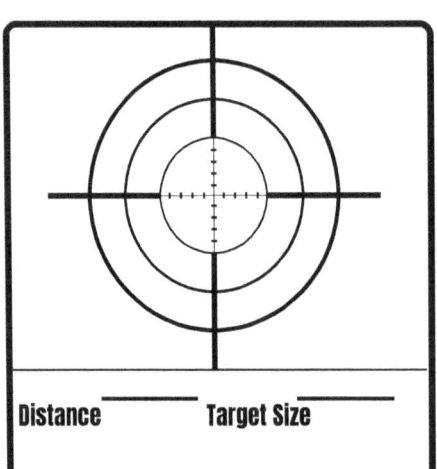

Distance _____ Target Size _____

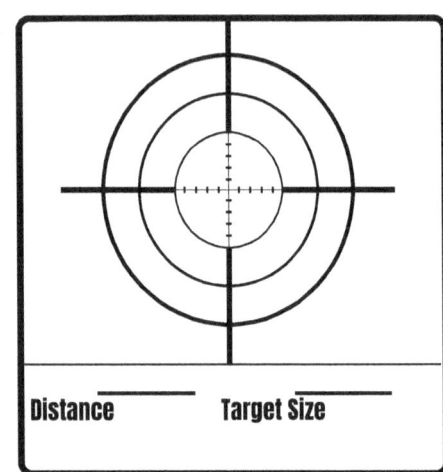

Distance _____ Target Size _____

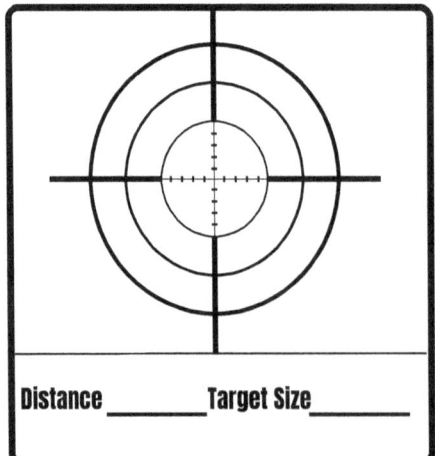

Distance _____ Target Size _____

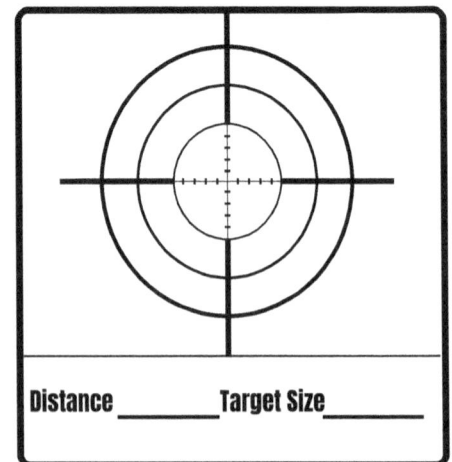

Distance _____ Target Size _____

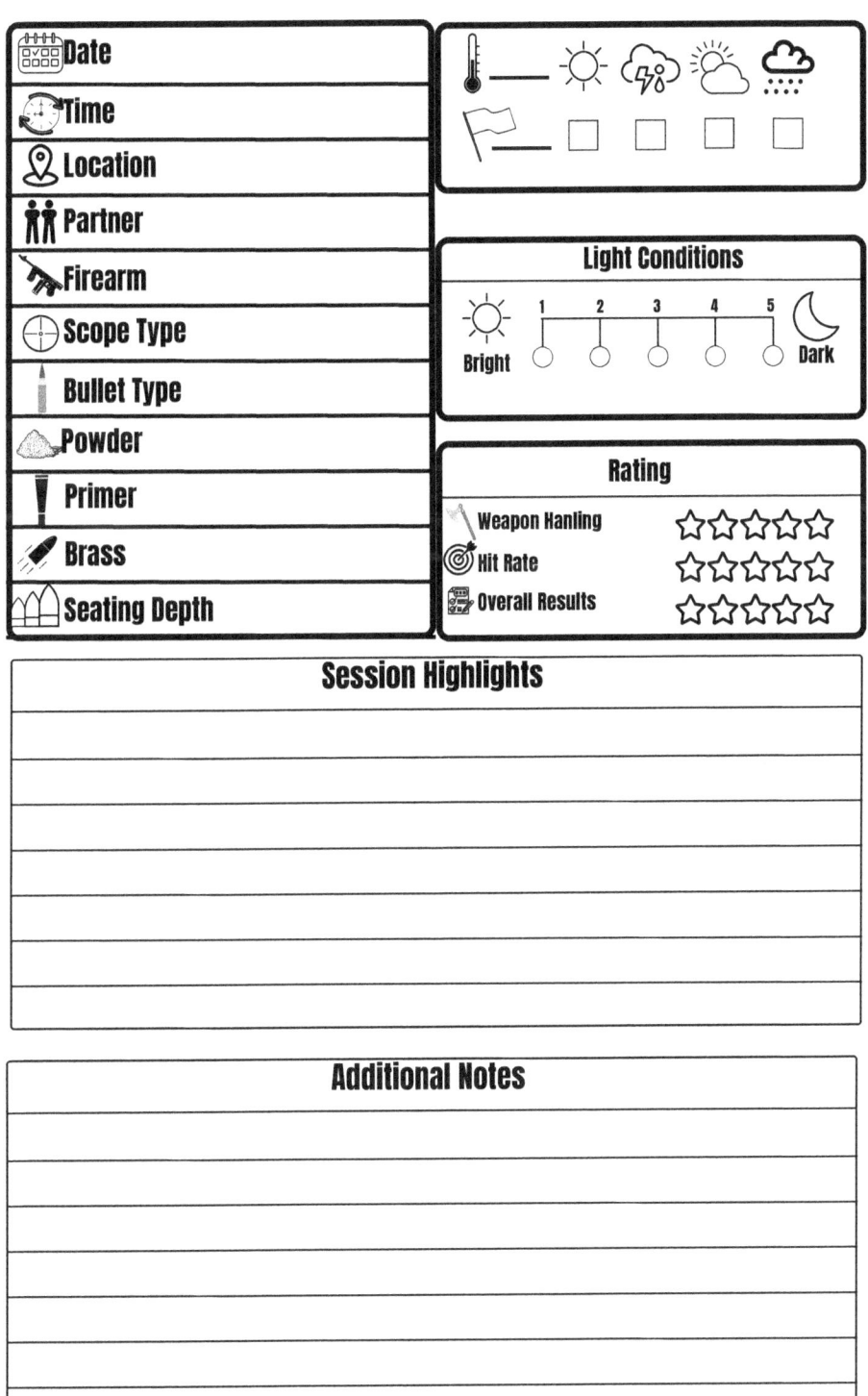

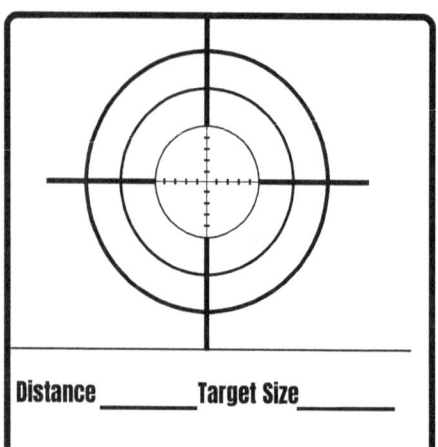

Distance _____ Target Size _____

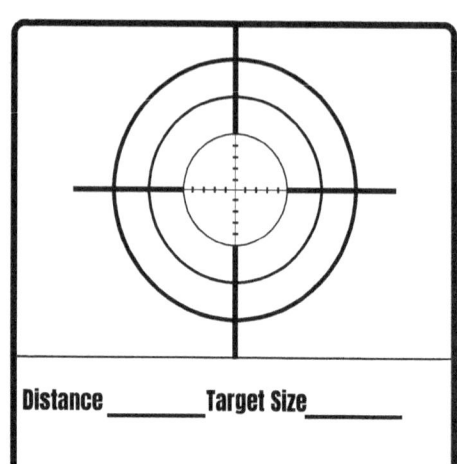

Distance _____ Target Size _____

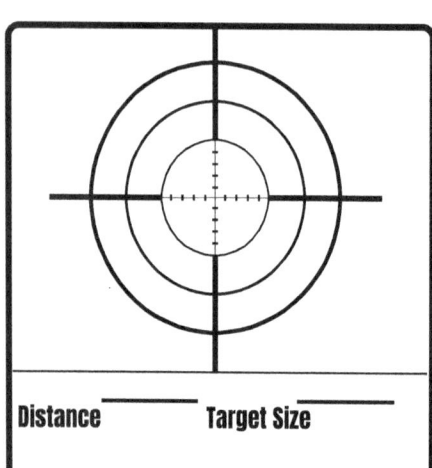

Distance _____ Target Size _____

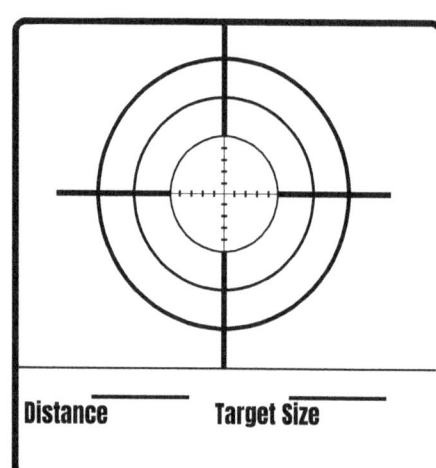

Distance _____ Target Size _____

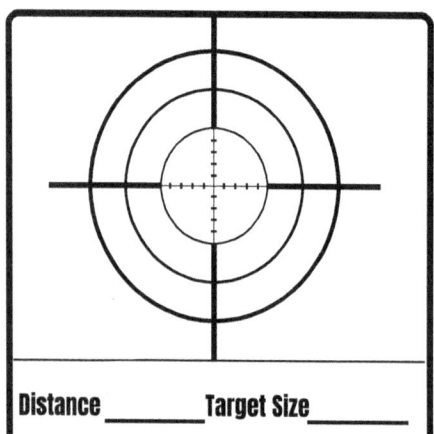

Distance _____ Target Size _____

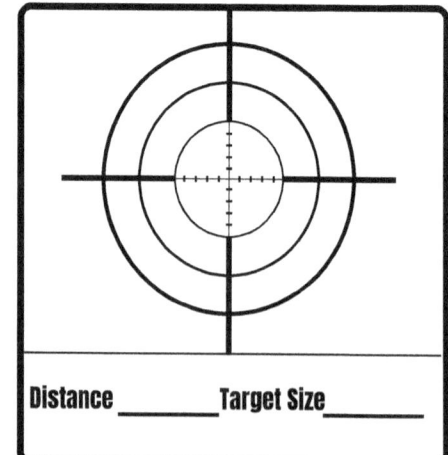

Distance _____ Target Size _____

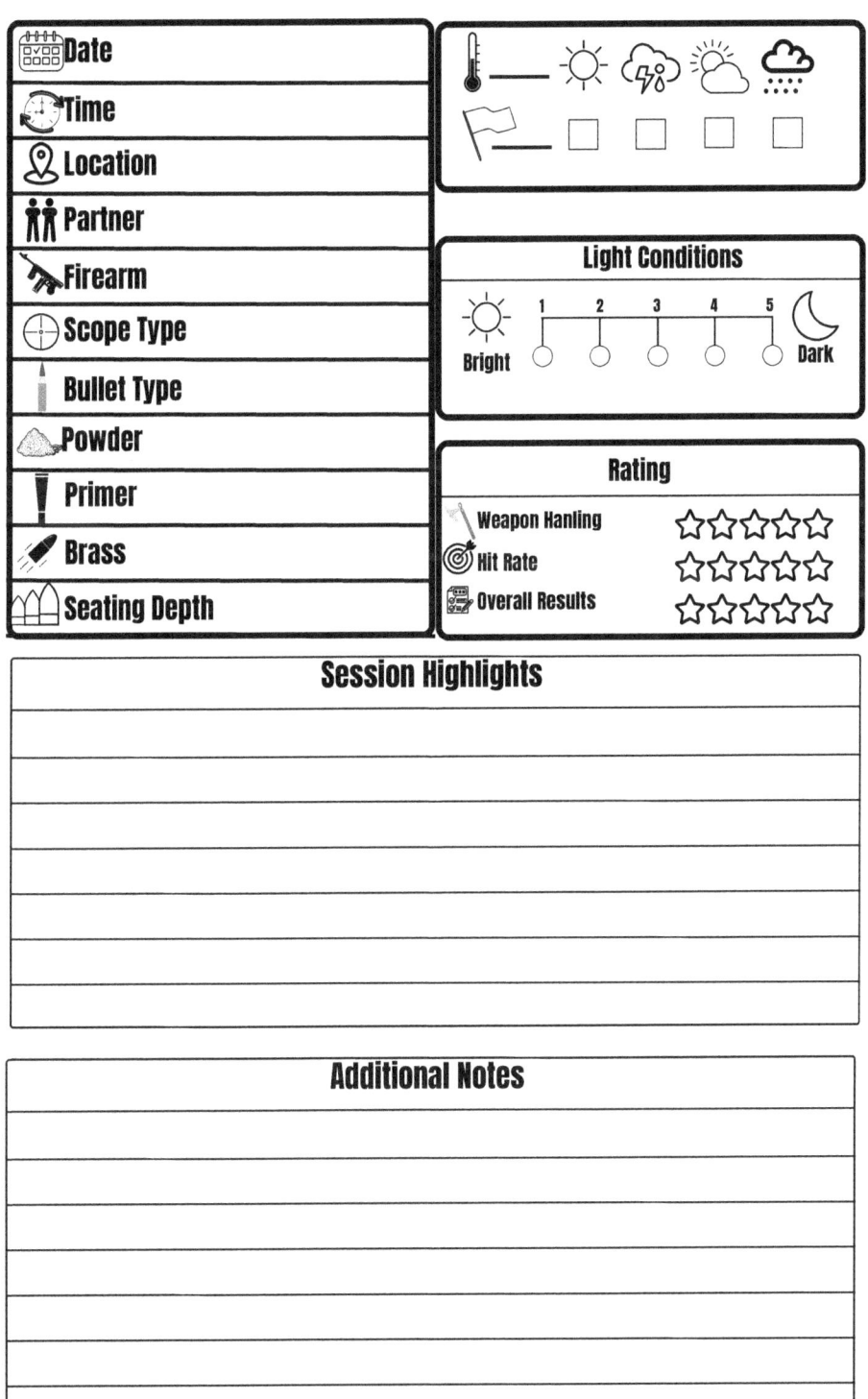

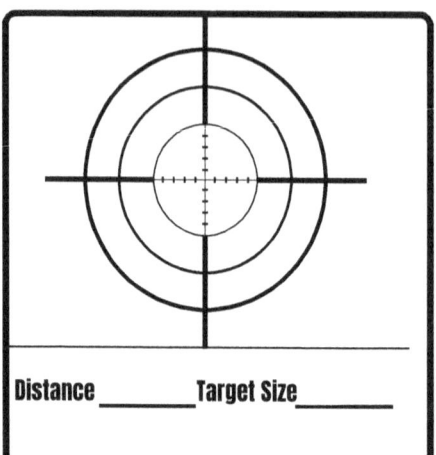
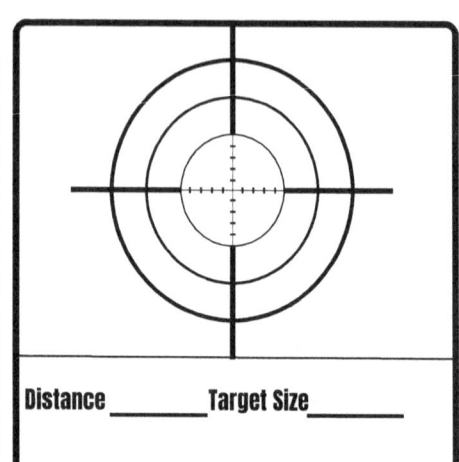
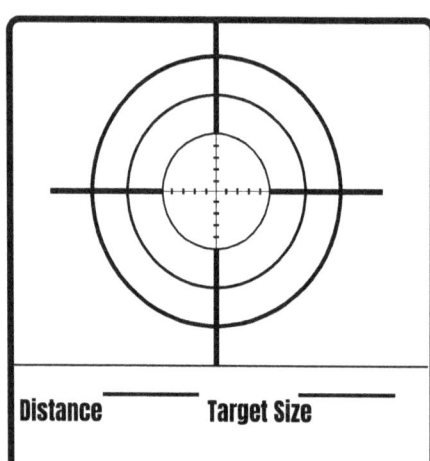
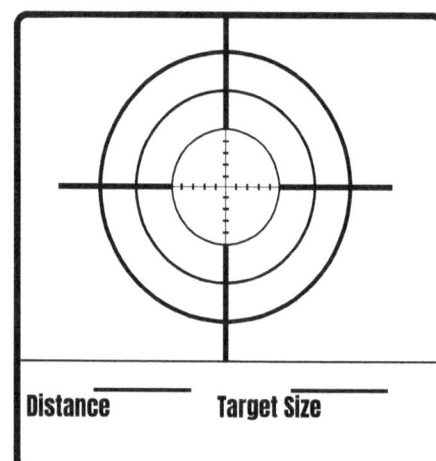
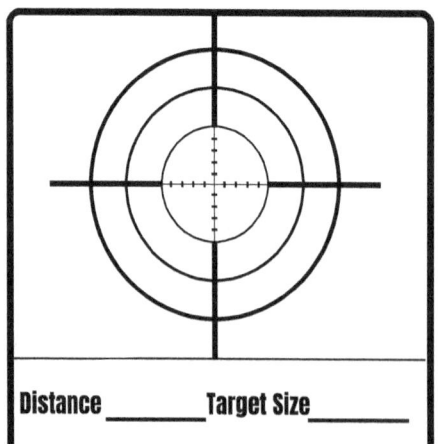
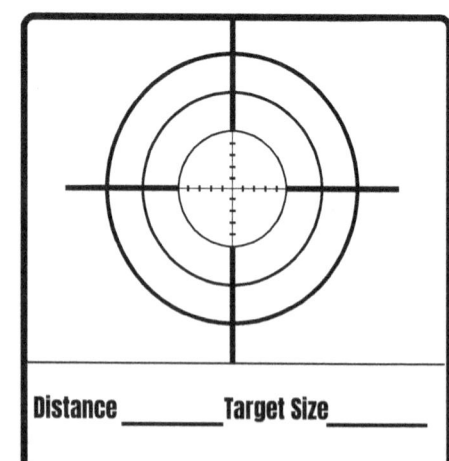

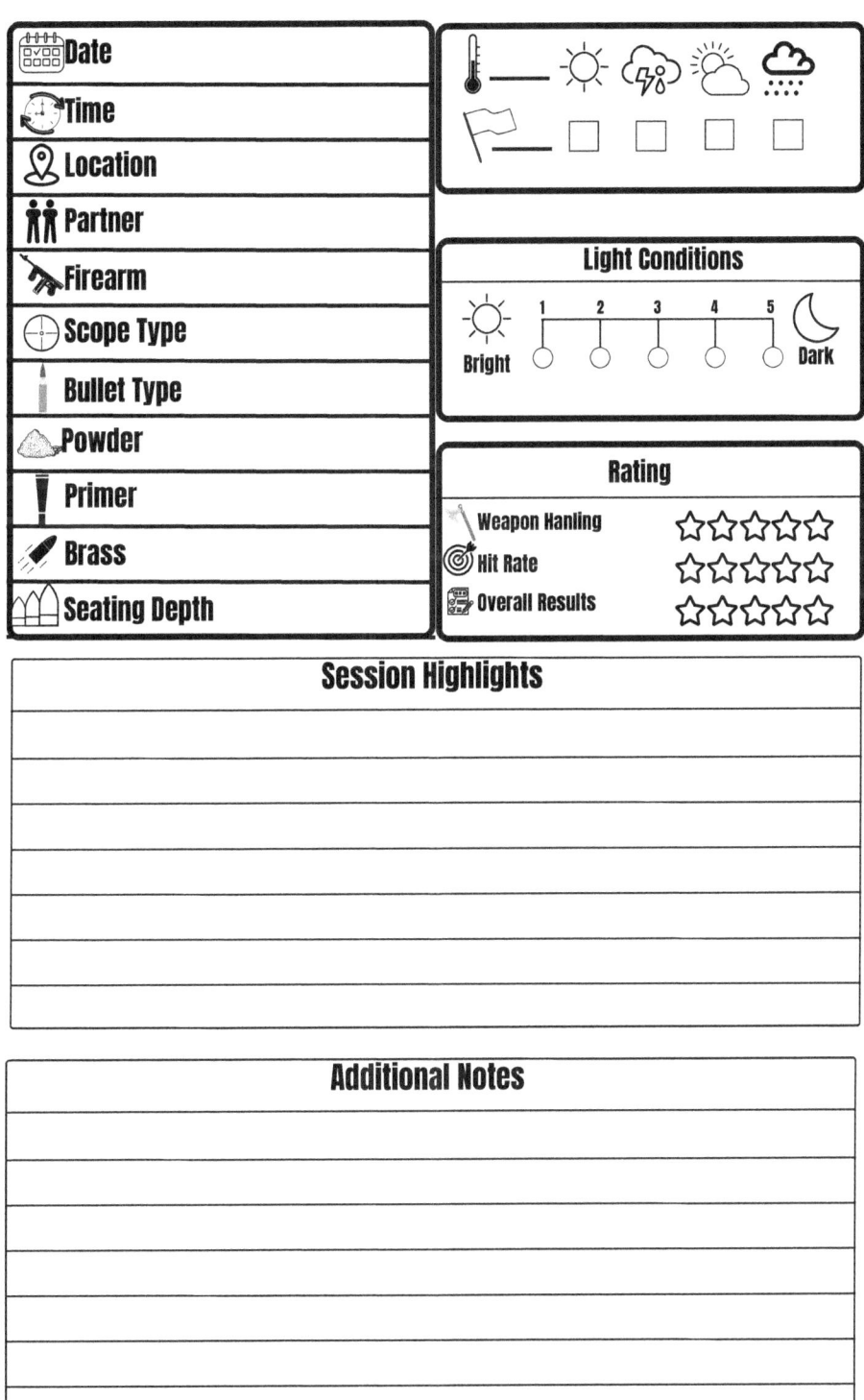

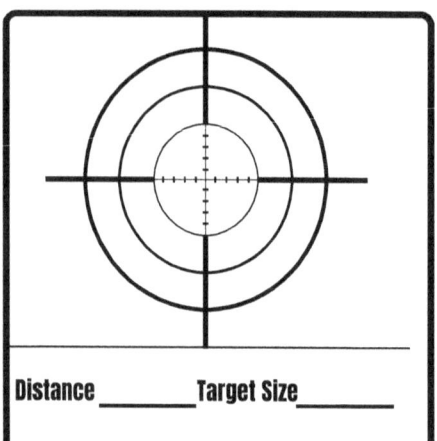
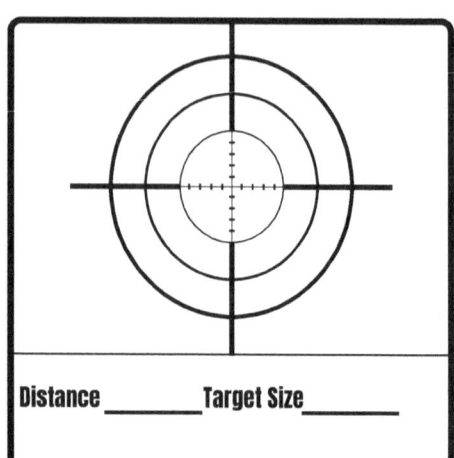
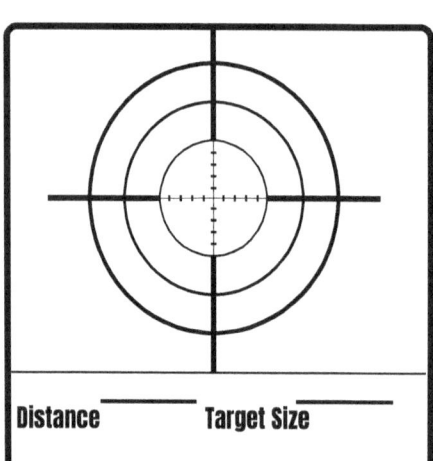
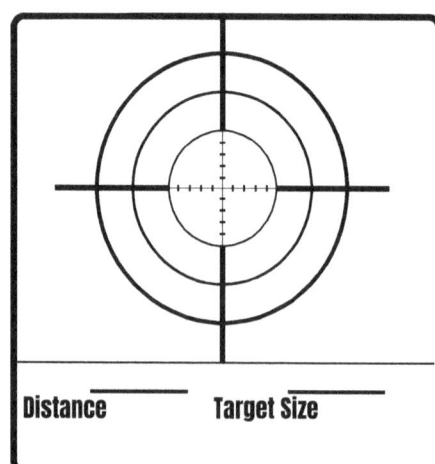
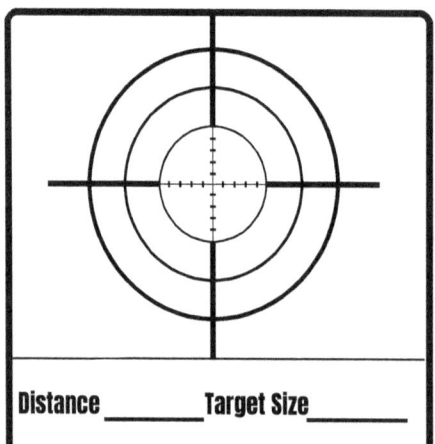
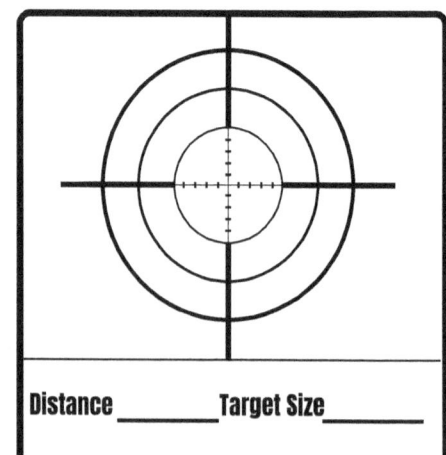

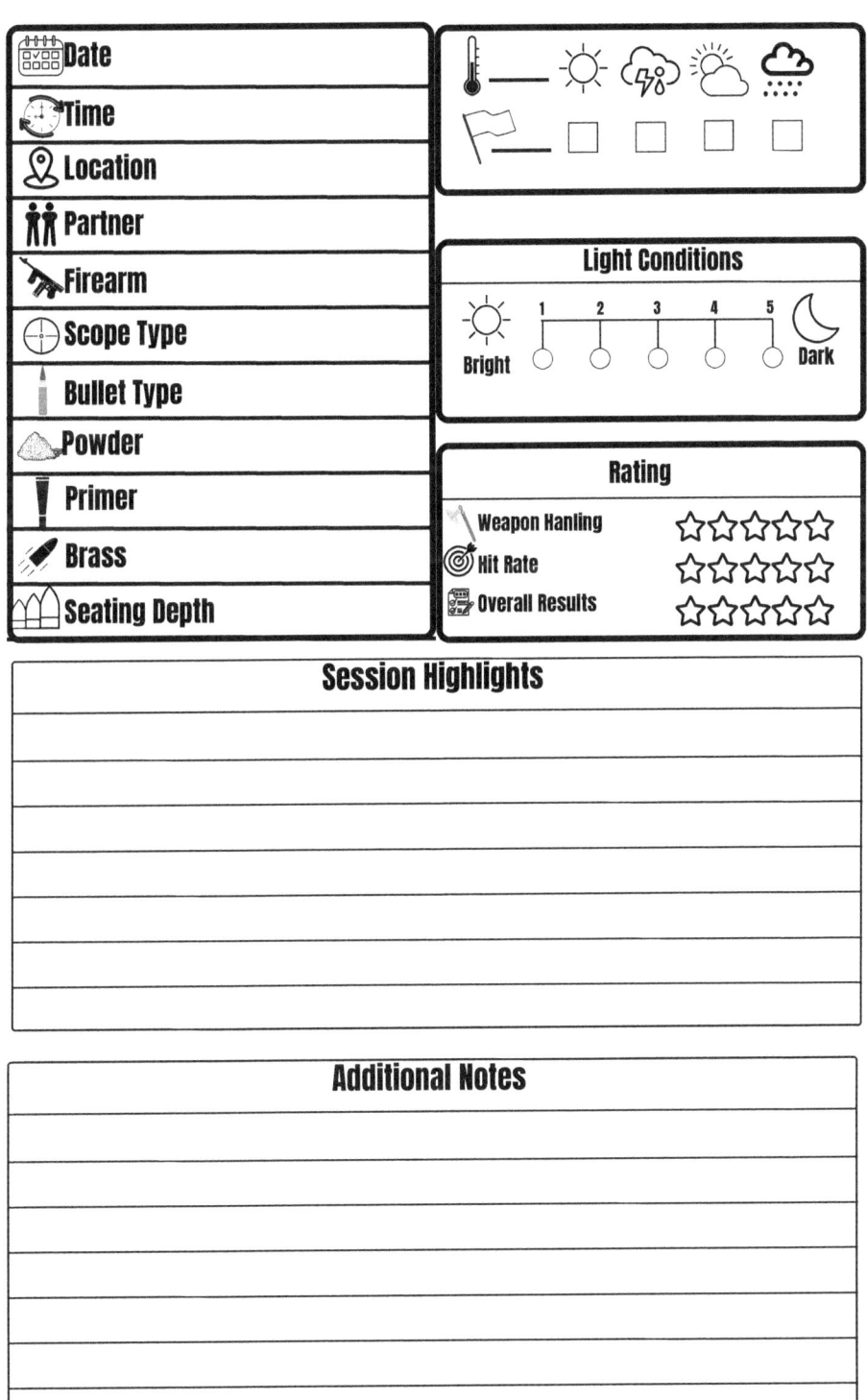

Session Highlights

Additional Notes

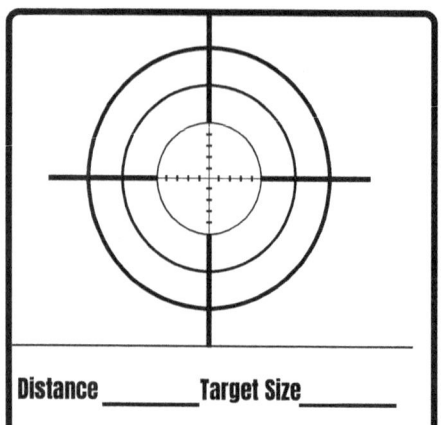

Distance _____ Target Size _____

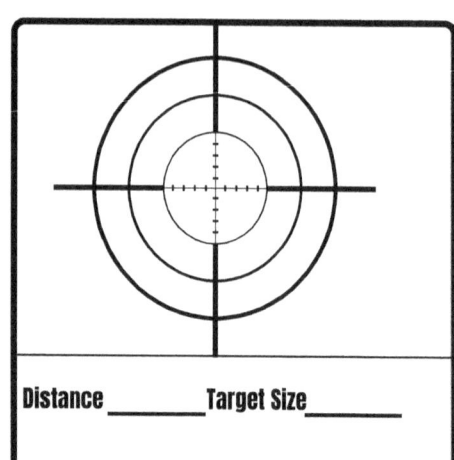

Distance _____ Target Size _____

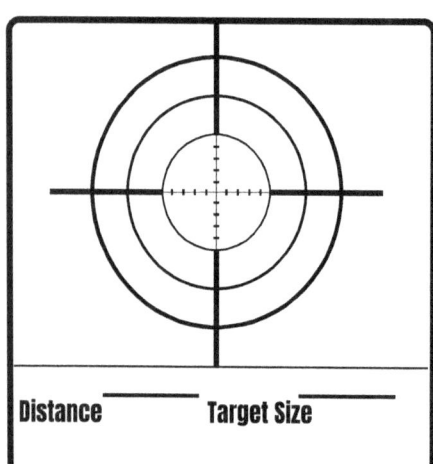

Distance _____ Target Size _____

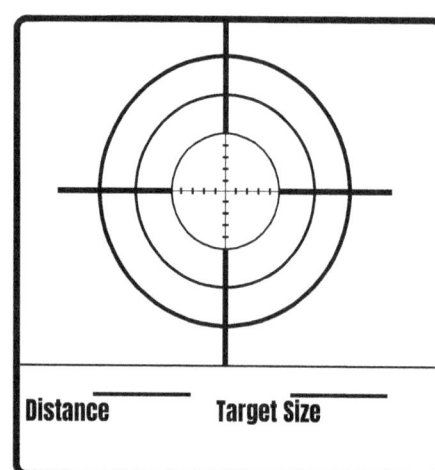

Distance _____ Target Size _____

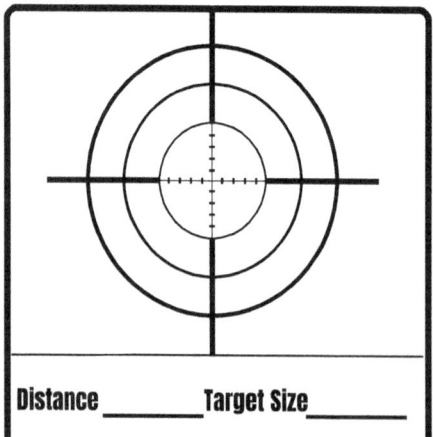

Distance _____ Target Size _____

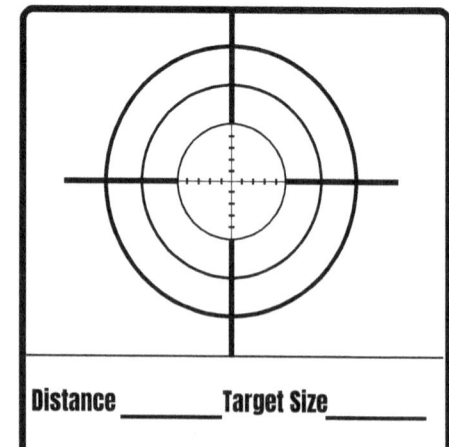

Distance _____ Target Size _____

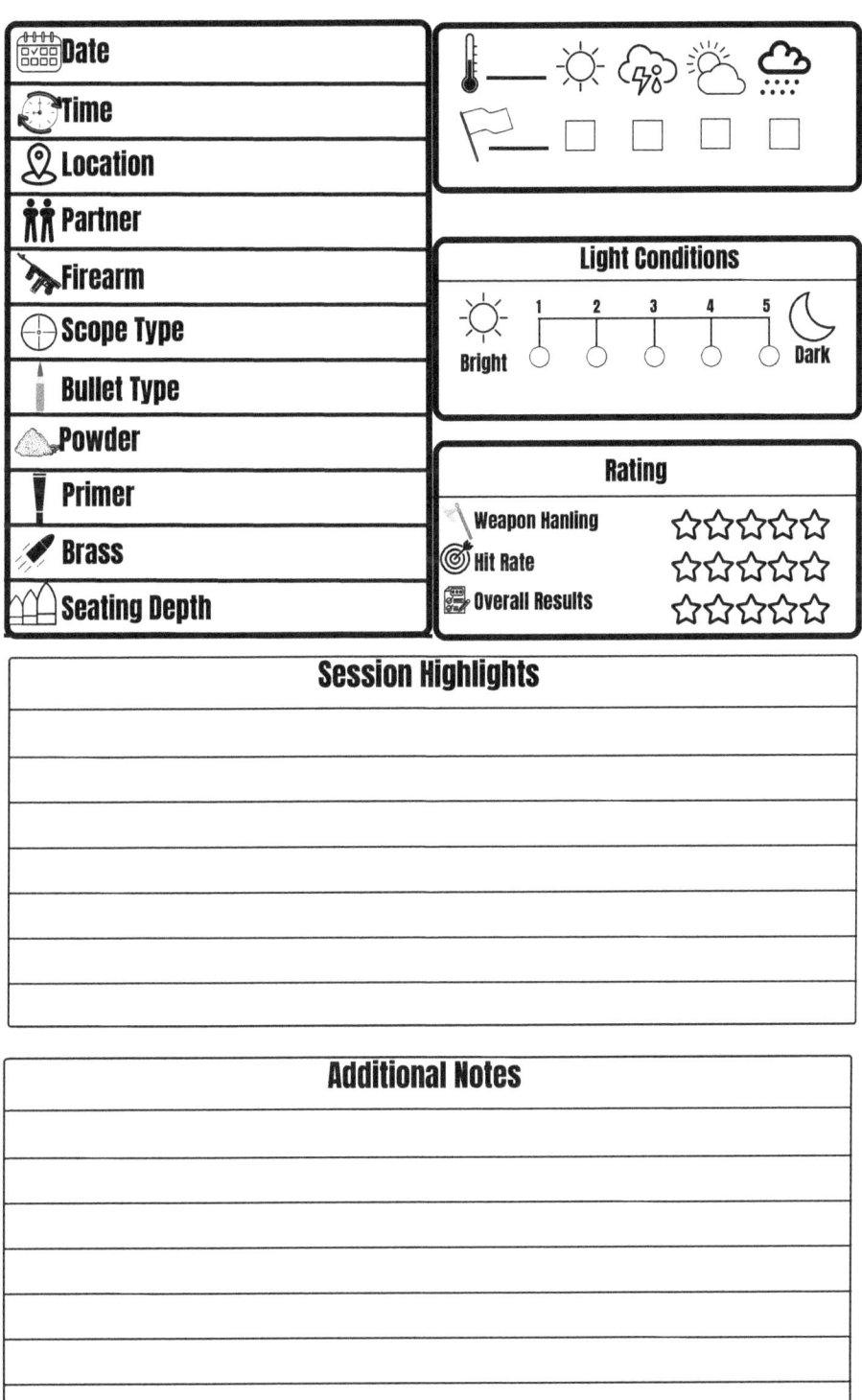

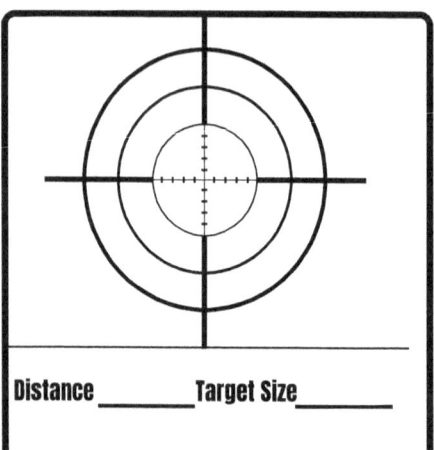

Distance _____ Target Size _____

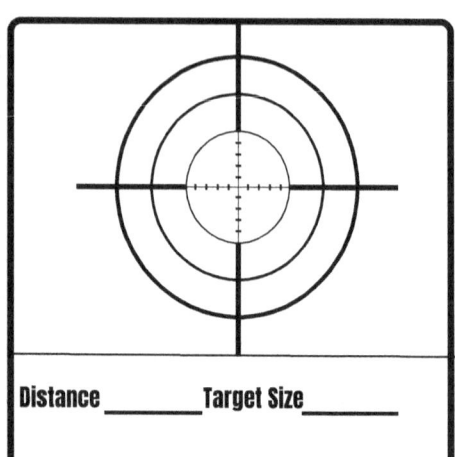

Distance _____ Target Size _____

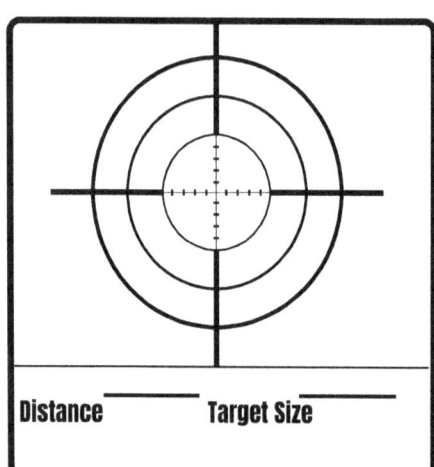

Distance _____ Target Size _____

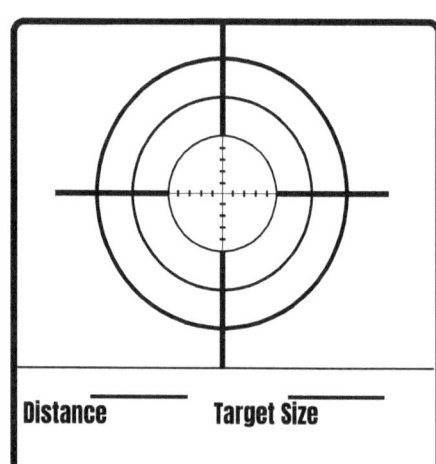

Distance _____ Target Size _____

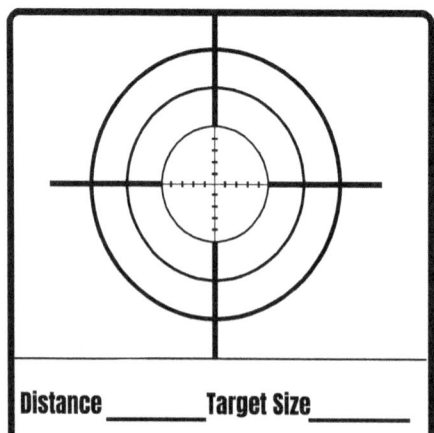

Distance _____ Target Size _____

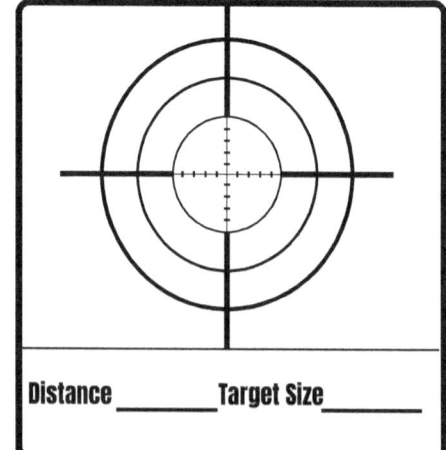

Distance _____ Target Size _____

Thank you!

WE ARE GLAD THAT YOU PURCHASED OUR BOOK!
PLEASE LET US KNOW HOW WE CAN IMPROVE IT!
YOUR FEEDBACK IS ESSENTIAL TO US.

Contact us at:

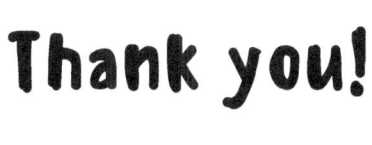 log'Sin@gmail.com

---

JUST TITLE THE EMAIL 'CREATIVE' AND WE WILL GIVE YOU SOME EXTRA SURPRISES!

www.ingramcontent.com/pod-product-compliance
Lightning Source LLC
Chambersburg PA
CBHW071003080526
44587CB00015B/2333